Keep Your Singing Voice Healthy!

Praise for *Keep Your Singing Voice Healthy!*

"This is the clearest explanation I have ever read of the basic mechanics and physiology of singing. The authors avoid any medical or scientific jargon, yet what they say checks out when read by someone who also knows that jargon. They put their extensive clinical experience at the service of the reader without ever claiming too much certainty and with constant respect for the variability of voices and circumstances. All the while, they don't try to make the book a substitute for a doctor or a voice teacher, a temptation not avoided by everyone who writes about these topics. Dr. Jahn and Dr. Cho are experts both musically and medically, and have the additional gift of writing in straightforward English, with a good sense of narrative and crystal-clear organization. Every singer should read what they have to say."

—**Will Crutchfield**, Conductor and Musicologist

"Navigating the often-treacherous journey of a singing career can be overwhelming, particularly as much of it is faced in isolation. Longevity requires expert guidance, even-handed information, and a thorough understanding of both the physiology and psychology of the singers. Drs. Jahn and Cho provide this in abundance with their comprehensive understanding of and hands-on expertise in how to take care of both our instruments and ourselves. Their book is a gift to anyone looking to deepen their understanding of the health of their voice."

—**Joyce DiDonato**, Multiple Grammy
Award–Winning Mezzo-soprano

"*Keep Your Singing Voice Healthy* by Drs. Jahn and Cho is inspiring and educational, and highly recommended for every singer interested in a long and healthy career."

—**Simon Estes**, Bass-baritone and Professor
of Vocal Pedagogy, Boston University

"This book provides a comprehensive exploration of the technical nuances of the singing voice, offering valuable insights into vocal mechanics. A must-read for anyone serious about refining their vocal skills."

—**Denyce Graves-Montgomery**, Mezzo-soprano, and Distinguished Visiting Faculty, The Juilliard School

"Knowledge is power, and the information so clearly laid out in this book will empower every singer to make the right decisions to maintain or improve their vocal health. Rooted in a deep understanding of the voice and of the professional demands of singers and their 'instrument,' Dr. Jahn and Dr. Cho's book is a welcome and long overdue resource."

—**Thomas Lausmann**, Director of Music Administration, The Metropolitan Opera

"Drs. Cho and Jahn have cared for the singers in the Metropolitan Opera chorus over many years now. We have relied on them to get us back to vocal health, and they have worked tirelessly to help keep artists performing at their highest level. Their book is a unique compendium of detailed information that every singer should read, absorb, and put into practice. It is a revelation to understand how much we can do for ourselves to maintain a healthy voice."

—**Donald Palumbo**, Chorus Master, The Metropolitan Opera

"As a performer on both the operatic and musical theater stages, I find this book presents an outstanding source of information about the singing voice. It is a must-read for singers and actors who seek a long professional career."

—**Paulo Szot**, Tony Award–Winning Baritone (*South Pacific*)

Keep Your Singing Voice Healthy!

The Doctor's Guide to Vocal Vitality and Longevity

ANTHONY F. JAHN, MD
YOUNGNAN JENNY CHO, MD

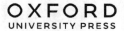

OXFORD
UNIVERSITY PRESS

Oxford University Press is a department of the University of Oxford.
It furthers the University's objective of excellence in research, scholarship,
and education by publishing worldwide. Oxford is a registered trade mark of
Oxford University Press in the UK and in certain other countries.

Published in the United States of America by Oxford University Press
198 Madison Avenue, New York, NY 10016, United States of America.

© Oxford University Press 2024
Illustrations © Mount Sinai Health System, Inc. Reprinted with
permission (unless otherwise noted).

All rights reserved. No part of this publication may be reproduced, stored in a retrieval system,
or transmitted, in any form or by any means, without the prior permission in writing of Oxford
University Press, or as expressly permitted by law, by license or under terms agreed with the
appropriate reprographics rights organization. Inquiries concerning reproduction outside the scope
of the above should be sent to the Rights Department, Oxford University Press, at the address above.

You must not circulate this work in any other form and you must
impose this same condition on any acquirer

CIP data is on file at the Library of Congress

ISBN 9780197629673 (pbk.)
ISBN 9780197629666 (hbk.)

DOI: 10.1093/9780197629703.001.0001

Paperback printed by Marquis Book Printing, Canada
Hardback printed by Bridgeport National Bindery, Inc., United States of America

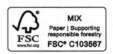

Contents

Preface	ix
1. The Vocal Apparatus	1
2. From Function to Performance	21
3. Examining Your Instrument: A Hands-On Tour	31
4. Monitoring Your Voice	37
5. The Glissando Test: A Simple Vocal Checkup	41
6. Hearing and Singing	45
7. Muscle Tension and the Voice	51
8. Frequent Complaints, Common-Sense Solutions	74
9. A Practical Approach to Allergies	98
10. Visiting the Voice Doctor	105
11. Common Disorders of the Larynx	114
12. Vitamins, Supplements, and Medications	129
13. Alcohol, Coffee, and Tobacco	139
14. Cortisone and the Voice	144
15. Voice Rest	150
16. Mindful Practice: A Medical Perspective	157

viii CONTENTS

17. Diet and Singing 163

18. Exercise and Vocal Health 172

19. The Living Instrument: The Voice over Time 176

20. The Singer: Artist and Artisan 182

Appendix 1: Ten Simple Tips for Keeping Your Voice Healthy 185
Appendix 2: Anatomic Intermezzo: What Do You Call
    That Thing? 187
Index 193

Preface

Many books have been written for singers. Their approach usually reflects the teacher-student relationship. Our purpose here is different. As laryngologists, we would like to share with you our understanding of the voice from the medical point of view. We offer that information to empower you: it is your instrument, and you should be in possession of every bit of knowledge that allows you to take control of your voice. Knowledge sheds light on areas that are otherwise the domain of imagery and mythology. That need not be; you can own your voice in an active and hands-on way, and hopefully this book will guide you in this endeavor. And, although much of this advice may reflect a classical music perspective, it should be useful for all styles of singing.

But first, a brief disclaimer: Our suggestions, while hopefully helpful, are just suggestions. This book does not offer personal medical advice. Since, even for the most healthy and proactive singer, individualized medical intervention is at times necessary, we recommend that you consult your physician if your symptoms persist or worsen.

This book is addressed to singers at all levels and of all ages. We consider singing a lifelong pursuit, involving technical mastery of an ever-changing instrument and an unending exploration of the musical art. It is assumed that you have musicality and the desire to sing well. But talent is like potential energy. The bridge connecting aptitude to ability (and, ultimately, to accomplishment) is skill, derived from understanding, both theoretical and experiential, put into practice—and, of course, practice!

How to build that bridge? Most importantly, you need to focus, to cultivate an in-the-moment awareness that connects you to your instrument, your body. Your voice is your best teacher if you listen to it. You are the master of your voice, and it is the purpose of this book to help singers take full ownership of their instrument and deal with the various factors, both extrinsic and intrinsic, that may affect singing over a lifetime.

It is our belief that a healthy voice comes from a healthy body. For this reason, we have included some suggestions for general health maintenance, dealing with subjects such as diet and exercise. You will also find that several points are repeated in various chapters. While some may reflect prevailing wisdom and others may seem novel, all are concepts we consider important to the rational management of vocal disorders. These should be your takeaway.

The ideas in this book reflect years of study and experience, discussions with voice teachers and speech therapists, much thought, and hundreds of nights spent at the Metropolitan Opera and other theaters. Our advice is also based on what we have learned from our patients, from the youngest beginners to the top professionals in the field. From them, we have gained a better understanding of the craft and a humbling appreciation of art. We thank them for what we have learned and would like to share this with you here.

Docendo discimus.

Anthony F. Jahn, MD
Youngnan Jenny Cho, MD

1

The Vocal Apparatus

The vocal apparatus can be divided into three main parts. The lungs, with the help of the diaphragm and the abdominal and pelvic muscles, provide the **power source** for moving air through the larynx. The vibrating vocal folds in the larynx are the **sound source**. And the upper part of the vocal tract, including the portions of the larynx above the vocal folds, the pharynx, the mouth, the tongue, the teeth, and the nasal and sinus cavities, form the **sound processors** of the voice.

The Power Source: Lungs and Abdomen

Although the larynx generates sound, the power comes from below. Air, drawn into the lungs and then expelled in a prolonged and controlled fashion, constitutes the fuel for the voice. The lungs are in the thorax, and as we breathe quietly, they normally fill and empty 12 to 16 times a minute. While the fully inflated lungs contain four to six liters of air (total lung capacity), we typically move three to five liters with each deep breath (vital capacity).

Air flows passively into the lungs as the thoracic cavity expands and then flows out as the thorax contracts. Although respiration is normally reflexive, it can of course also be consciously controlled, and good breath control is an essential part of singing. The rate of air flow during singing is regulated by balancing the upward pressure exerted by the abdominal muscles against the glottic resistance exerted by the contraction of the vocal folds above.

Keep Your Singing Voice Healthy! Anthony F. Jahn and Youngnan Jenny Cho, Oxford University Press.
© Oxford University Press 2024. DOI: 10.1093/9780197629703.003.0001

2   KEEP YOUR SINGING VOICE HEALTHY!

The thoracic cavity inflates in two ways (Figure 1.1). The intercostal muscles lift the 12 ribs and expand the chest outward. The effect is like raising and lowering 12 bucket handles that are linked to each other. When the ribs are raised during inspiration, the thoracic cavity expands in a horizontal (or transverse) direction, as the cross section of the chest changes from oval to more circular. When we breathe out, the ribs are lowered down again, and the intrathoracic volume contracts. This is called **thoracic breathing**. While thoracic breathing is normal for some people, it is rather labor intensive, does not fully expand the thoracic cavity, and is not adequate for the needs of the singer.

A second method, **abdominal breathing**, involves the diaphragm and the abdominal muscles. Abdominal breathing expands the thoracic cavity in a vertical direction and is more effective than thoracic breathing, moving a greater volume of air with less effort. The diaphragm consists of two thin, oval dome–like sheets of muscle, which separate the thorax above from the abdomen below. It forms the floor of the thoracic "bird cage." During inhalation the diaphragm contracts and the domes pull down and flatten, lowering the floor of the thoracic cavity and drawing air into the lungs. During passive exhalation, the diaphragm muscle relaxes, and the contents of the abdomen push it up, expelling air from the lungs.

Exhalation is normally also reflexive, but when used to power the voice, it can be actively enhanced. By purposely contracting the muscles of the abdomen and tightening the floor of the pelvis, the contents of the abdomen are pushed up toward the chest with greater force and efficiency. Since active exhalation and phonation occur when the diaphragm is relaxed, the concept of "singing from the diaphragm" is misleading, and probably meant to direct the singer's attention to the lower ribs and the breastbone (sternum), where the anterior abdominal muscles insert and contract during phonation. Singing from the diaphragm actually occurs with a relaxed diaphragm, and it may be only a slight overstatement to say that the singer's main power source is the abdomen.

THE VOCAL APPARATUS   3

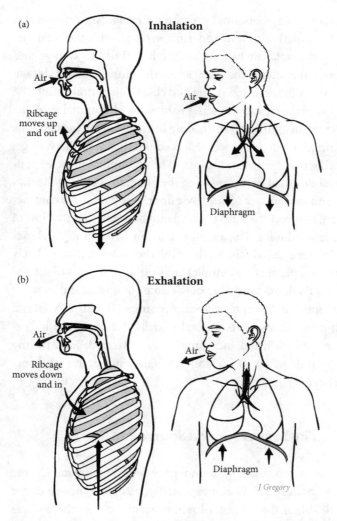

Figure 1.1 The two phases of breathing: During inhalation, the rib cage lifts and the diaphragm descends, expanding the chest cavity. With exhalation, the rib cage drops down and the diaphragm rises, forcing air out of the lungs.

4 KEEP YOUR SINGING VOICE HEALTHY!

To visualize the abdominal breathing mechanism more easily, we might compare it to a hypodermic syringe, with the rigid air-containing thoracic cavity forming the barrel of the syringe and the abdominal contents the plunger. As the plunger is withdrawn, negative pressure is created in the barrel, and air is drawn into the syringe: the diaphragm contracts, pushing the abdominal contents down. When the plunger is pushed up into the barrel, the contents of the syringe, air in this case, are forced out the tip of the syringe, representing the trachea and larynx. The abdominal muscles constrict the abdominal cavity, pushing the viscera up against the diaphragm, and the muscles of the pelvic floor simultaneously contract and stiffen, to direct the push upward into the chest and the flow of air past the vocal folds. The analogy is of course not completely accurate, since the barrel (the walls of the thorax) is not completely rigid, and the "plunger" is definitely not rigid—the walls of the abdomen and its floor, consisting of the anterior and lateral muscles of the abdomen and the pelvic floor, all contract during exhalation.

For singers, the use of abdominal muscles during controlled exhalation must be learned and consciously cultivated, since during normal "untrained" quiet breathing, inhalation is active while exhalation occurs passively.

The Larynx: Sound Source and More

The larynx is the primary sound generator in humans. If any structure vibrates rapidly and repeatedly, turbulent air waves are produced. When the rate of vibration occurs within the audible range (which is about 20 to 20,000 times per second), those air waves can stimulate the inner ear, and we hear it as sound. There are of course many other sound generators in the animal kingdom, as diverse as the forewing of a cricket or the syrinx of a bird. Neither of these animals has a larynx such as ours, and neither uses vocal folds to make a sound. Like us, however, they have taken a preexisting

THE VOCAL APPARATUS 5

anatomic structure that originally evolved for a different purpose and secondarily adapted it to make sound.

What, then, is the primary function of the larynx? In humans, as in all mammals, it is to protect the airway. Breathing and swallowing share a common pathway in the lower pharynx, and as we breathe or swallow, it is important that inhaled air and ingested food each go to their proper destination.

It is difficult to overestimate the vital protective role of the larynx in this regard. If the airway were not shielded during a swallow, food and liquids would be aspirated into the lungs, resulting in pneumonia and possibly death. It is for this reason that the larynx has evolved not merely as a simple valve but as a *triple* sphincter, which reflexively and firmly closes the airway during swallow, allowing the food or liquid to continue into the esophagus and the stomach. These three sphincters, or valves, consist of (1) the epiglottis and aryepiglottic folds, (2) the false vocal folds, and finally (3) the true vocal folds. The first two are supraglottic (above the vocal folds), while the last, and most important, is the glottis itself, the opening between the vocal folds.

In addition to triple closure, during a swallow the larynx is pulled up and forward, moving it out of the way of the swallowed bolus. This not only further protects the airway but also opens the back of the hypopharynx and the entrance to the esophagus. Conceptually, this is like throwing a switch on the railroad track, directing "the train" (whether a breath of air or a gulp of food) to travel to its appropriate destination.

The elevation and forward movement of the larynx involves several sets of "levator" muscles. Once the swallow is complete, the larynx is returned to its lower and more posterior breathing position by another set of "depressor" muscles. There are eight muscles that elevate the larynx, far greater in number and strength than the two depressor muscles, once again underscoring its significance as guardian of the airway. When a swallow is initiated, the rapid closure, elevation, and anterior displacement of the larynx, followed

6 KEEP YOUR SINGING VOICE HEALTHY!

by its slower reset when the swallow is complete, are entirely involuntary. One step follows the other, in a reflexive chain of events.

There are two other laryngeal functions we should consider before getting to voice production. Cough is an important mechanism that rapidly clears the airway of debris. It is also typically reflexive, although it can be initiated voluntarily. A cough is usually triggered by irritation of the larynx, trachea, and bronchi. At the start of a cough, the vocal folds are momentarily firmly squeezed together, while intrathoracic air pressure builds up. The laryngeal muscles then release, and the folds suddenly fly apart, as air is explosively expelled from the lower respiratory tract. During a cough, the airflow may be as high as 70 miles per hour, reaching almost hurricane speeds. The blast of wind carries with it excess mucus, inhaled foreign material, and any other irritant. A productive cough, one that clears infected mucus from the lungs, is an important part of normal recovery following a respiratory infection.

Finally, we can voluntarily squeeze the larynx shut for longer periods of time, to build up pressure in the chest and abdomen. This move, the Valsalva maneuver, has several important uses. By holding our breath, we can stiffen the chest wall, allowing our muscles to brace against the ribcage and work more effectively, as when we lift or carry a heavy object. Immobilizing the chest also allows contracting abdominal muscles to direct their effort downward, toward the pelvis. This is important when we bear down on the toilet and during childbirth.

Despite all that has been written about it, the untrained larynx is really a mechanical device with a rather limited repertoire: it can open and close (abduction or adduction), it can be raised or lowered (elevation or depression), and the vocal folds can passively vibrate as air flows past them. What makes the larynx interesting as a sound source is the degree of sophistication with which these simple actions have been co-opted for voice production, and the ability of the singer to separate and gain voluntary control over

THE VOCAL APPARATUS 7

the different steps of what is normally a mass reflex. Hidden in the reflexive movements of the untrained larynx lie some of the basic tools of vocal technique. The muscles closing the vocal folds control pitch, the muscles modifying the shape of the supraglottic compartments affect resonance and quality, and the balance between vocal fold tension and subglottic air pressure is involved in volume. This balanced coordination of the respiratory muscles in producing efficient vocal sounds is the definition of *appoggio*.

It is interesting (although somewhat idle) to speculate how the first vocal utterance might have occurred. Was it during extreme effort, when the vocal folds were inadvertently forced apart and set into vibration? Was it during a moment of extreme stress or excitement when forceful breathing became audible? Was it a grunt, meant to clear the vocal tract of foreign matter? In any case, over time vocal sounds, with variations in rhythm, loudness, and pitch, became more prolonged, varied, and sophisticated. Vocal communication, progressing to speech and song, began.

The larynx is a structure with a rigid framework that contains numerous moving parts (Figure 1.2). Its walls are formed by the **thyroid cartilage** above and the **cricoid cartilage** below. The thyroid cartilage, shaped like the keel of a ship, is open in the back. It sits atop the signet ring–shaped cricoid cartilage and is hinged posteriorly, so it can tilt forward and backward like the visor on a helmet. The cricoid cartilage is a complete ring, and rigid. The paired smaller L-shaped **arytenoid cartilages** are perched on the upper rim of the posterior cricoid and project into the airway. They are attached to the vocal folds and are highly mobile: they can tilt, swivel, and move together and apart. Above, the larynx is suspended by muscles from the **hyoid bone**, at the base of the tongue. Below, it sits on top of the trachea. Internally, the larynx is covered by the **epiglottis**, which looks somewhat like a toilet lid. During swallow, the epiglottis flips down to cover the entrance to the larynx. The epiglottis is not involved in sound production and plays no role in speech or singing.

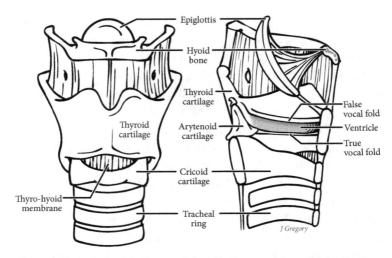

Figure 1.2 A view of the larynx from the front and in cross section. Note how the true vocal folds straddle the glottic opening, attached anteriorly to the inner surface of the cricoid cartilage and posteriorly to the mobile arytenoid cartilages.

All the active movements of the larynx are brought about by muscles both inside and outside the laryngeal framework. Most of these muscles are paired and work in an agonist-antagonist arrangement: if the muscles that close the laryngeal opening contract, the muscles that open the laryngeal inlet relax, and vice versa. In this, the arrangement is like muscles elsewhere in the body: when the biceps (which flexes your arm) contracts, the triceps (which extends the arm) relaxes.

Sound is produced as the vocal folds vibrate passively, in response to air flowing past them. The folds are attached in the front to the inside of the thyroid cartilage and come together at the anterior commissure. Posteriorly, each vocal fold is attached to one of the arytenoid cartilages. As these cartilages come together, move apart, or swivel, the V-shaped glottic aperture between the vocal folds is opened or closed.

THE VOCAL APPARATUS 9

During phonation, the folds are approximated in the midline by the laryngeal muscles and held in that position as air pressure below builds up (Figure 1.3). When air pressure is greater than vocal fold tension, the folds are momentarily forced apart. A burst of air from below is released and rushes past the edges of the vocal folds, setting them into vibration. Subglottic air pressure now

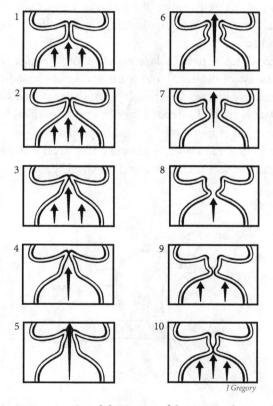

Figure 1.3 A cross-sectional depiction of the mucosal wave shows how vocal folds vibrate. Viewed from above (with a laryngoscope), the appearance is that of a gentle back-and-forth movement. Note how the edges oscillate in two segments, first the lower "lip" and then the upper "lip."

drops, the adductor muscles reassert themselves, the vocal folds reapproximate in the midline, and subglottic air pressure again builds up. The cycle is repeated hundreds of times each second (in the case of a soprano's high C, 1,046 times!), and the resultant intermittent release of "packets" of air creates the necessary stimulus for the listening ear—sound is produced. The flow of air sets the vocal folds into vibration, and sustained phonation creates a regular oscillation of the folds, called the mucosal wave. Different sets of muscles are involved in approximating the vocal folds, depending on the register.

The vocal folds have a layered structure (Figure 1.4). The bulk, or **body**, of the vocal fold is formed by the **vocalis muscle**, which is covered by an adherent layer of collagen, the **vocal ligament**. Overlying the ligament is a thin and more pliable mucous membrane (the superficial laryngeal epithelium), which forms the loosely attached **cover**. A slippery interface, **Reinke's space**, separates the surface membrane and the vocal ligament.

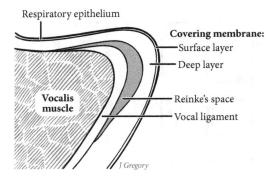

Figure 1.4 Cross-sectional structure of the vocal fold. The covering membrane is separated from the body of the vocal fold (vocal ligament and vocalis muscle) by Reinke's space, a slippery interface that is lubricated by hyaluronic acid gel. This allows the surface layer to vibrate separately when the deep layer is tightened, as in head voice.

THE VOCAL APPARATUS 11

The term Reinke's "space" is somewhat misleading: there is no actual physical space, but rather a separation between the vocal ligament and covering membrane. This contains a minuscule amount of hyaluronic acid, a viscous gel that is similar to the lubricating fluid in our joints. The slippery interface between the thin vocal membrane and the underlying vocal muscle allows the covering membrane to vibrate somewhat independently in response to expelled air.

When, during higher-pitched phonation, the "body" of the vocal fold is pulled taut, the "cover" becomes further disengaged, slipping and sliding with ever more freedom in response to the flow of air. In the highest range, only the very edge of the vocal fold vibrates, completely decoupled from the tightly held underlying vocal muscle.

Although the larynx is a complex anatomic structure, there is very little to distinguish the human larynx from those of other mammals. As we look at the video monitor, mesmerized by stroboscopic images of the vocal folds doing their gentle hula dance, it is sobering to consider that the vocal folds of a pig are visually indistinguishable from ours. Although undeniably the source of vocal sound, the essence of what makes our voice, whether speaking or singing, human does not reside in what the great mezzo Marilyn Horne referred to as "those two little bits of gristle."

The Upper Vocal Tract: Resonators and Processors

The raw sound that first emerges from the larynx is not pretty, and certainly nothing we would buy a ticket to hear. It is a bleating, quacking sound that resembles the sound of a party noisemaker or a kazoo. It has pitch and some power, but not much else. In fact, almost everything we prize in a well-trained musical voice is created in the upper vocal tract, which includes the air spaces above the larynx, the pharynx, the nose, and the mouth. This upper

12   KEEP YOUR SINGING VOICE HEALTHY!

vocal tract is a complex set of cavities that amplifies, refines, and imparts color, quality, and musical finesse to the naive sound of the fluttering vocal folds.

The main function of the upper vocal tract is amplification of the laryngeal sound. Of course, that sound is additionally modified by the articulators, the lips, tongue, and teeth, which integrate words into what would otherwise be only a *vocalise*, but it is the resonating function of the upper vocal tract that converts sound into voice. How does this come about?

Sympathetic vibration is a well-known physical phenomenon whereby a structure, such as a tuning fork or a string, can be set to vibrate by sound waves from a distant sound source. The concept of **resonance** here refers to the tendency of an enclosed air space to vibrate at characteristic and specific frequencies, defined by the size, shape, and degree of enclosure of the air cavity. If you have ever blown across the top of an empty bottle to make a sound, you are familiar with this phenomenon.

The acoustics of resonators were classically described by the German physicist Hermann Helmholtz (1821–1894). In his early experiments, he used empty rectangular wooden boxes that were set to vibrate with tuning forks (Figure 1.5). When the tuning fork of a certain frequency was attached to a box of a certain size and was activated, a marked amplification of the sound occurred. He found that any air-containing cavity had a specific resonant frequency that depended on its size. He further discovered that if the box was fully closed or open at one end, the contained air would vibrate at either one-half or one-quarter of the wavelength of the presented sound. What this means is that a fully enclosed resonating cavity will resonate one octave higher than a cavity that is open on one end. And this just describes the fundamental frequency—the harmonics, whole-number multiples of the fundamental, are also amplified, although to a lesser degree. Further experiments, using a resonating tube, have shown that any air-containing cavity, whether open or closed at either end, will resonate at several characteristic

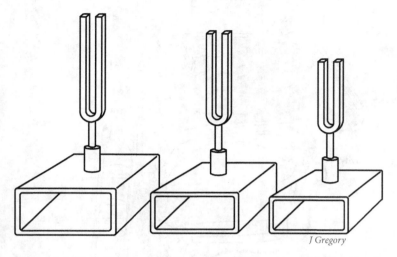

Figure 1.5 Helmholtz resonators. Each box contains a volume of air that resonates at the same frequency as the tuning fork and amplifies the sound.

frequencies, corresponding to a fundamental and its harmonics, thereby amplifying those sounds.

It then stands to reason that, by constantly changing the dimensions of a resonating air cavity, it is possible to amplify almost any sound. And this is what happens in the upper vocal tract. In this sense, the acoustic mechanism of the human voice perhaps most resembles the trombone. With the trombone, the sound source (the buzz generated by the player's lips) activates air vibration in the instrument. As the player moves the slide, he changes the resonant frequency of the trombone to change the pitch of the note the instrument plays.

Of course, to compare the upper vocal tract to a set of rectangular and rigid wooden boxes, or even a trombone, is overly simplistic. Every cavity in the upper vocal tract has its own dimensions and shape, whether the laryngeal ventricles right above the vocal folds, the pharynx, the nose, or the mouth (Figure 1.6). The contours

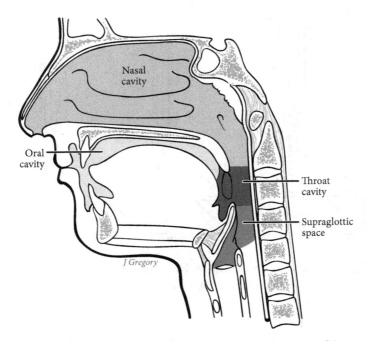

Figure 1.6 Sagittal section of the vocal tract, showing some of the resonating cavities above the larynx. These vary in size from the smallest (laryngeal ventricles) to the largest (pharynx).

and acoustic properties of these various cavities are complex and, unlike Helmholtz resonators, cannot be described by a simple formula. Furthermore, the walls enclosing these resonating cavities are lined by mucous membrane and may be soft or firm, reflective or absorptive, fixed or mobile; the air spaces may be small or large, variably shaped, fully open or partially closed—all factors that further modify resonance. In fact, by constantly moving the "baffles" that define these resonating spaces, the singer can readily modify the voice.

The resonant spaces in the upper vocal tract have a complex effect on the voice. First, by amplifying the fundamental frequency of raw laryngeal sound, they greatly increase overall loudness. But

THE VOCAL APPARATUS   15

by also selectively enhancing certain frequencies over others, the resonators can control the harmonic spectrum of the voice. By strengthening the higher overtones, for example, the voice may sound more incisive or nasal, whereas by emphasizing the lower harmonics, the voice becomes darker and warmer. Consider by comparison an instrument such as the oboe, which is readily identifiable by the nasality of its harmonic spectrum and rich in high-frequency overtones, versus a French horn, with a different harmonic spectrum emphasizing the lower harmonics.

Of specific interest are the laryngeal ventricles, the smallest resonators. These two niches are located just above the vocal folds and separate them from the false vocal folds. They resonate at a very high frequency (2,700 Hertz) and are believed to be responsible for the "singer's formant," a high overtone that distinguishes the singing voice and allows it to be heard over a loud orchestra. In other animals, such as some frogs and monkeys, laryngeal ventricles are larger and balloon out during phonation, forming a major amplifier for the voice.

And it is in these resonating spaces where the least appreciated (not to say "unsung") aspect of the technical virtuosity of the vocal performer lies. The moment-by-moment adjustments that are made in the upper vocal tract during singing, which change warmth, projection, and color, opening or covering the voice, in sum create the vocal signature of a specific singer and elude the sort of facile visual analysis that we have applied to the vibrating vocal folds.

The nose and sinuses are also part of the voice production, although in an indirect fashion. The nasal cavities may be considered as two hollow cylinders, open at both ends. In the front, the nostrils are defined by the soft cartilage of the nasal tip, while in the back, the two choanae open into the nasopharynx. These posterior openings are surrounded by bone and covered by thin mucous membrane, and their appearance is reminiscent of the McDonald's arches.

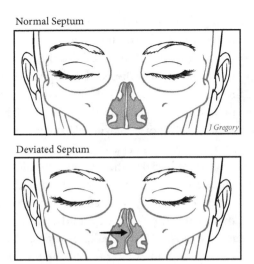

Figure 1.7 Deviation of the nasal septum, the partition separating the two nasal cavities, affects the resonant properties of the nose. When the problem is corrected, there is often improved resonance in the mask.

Nasal resonance is a function of the volume of air in each nasal cavity. This, in turn, is determined by the shape and position of the nasal septum separating the two cavities, and the size and shape of the turbinates, soft tissue–covered shelves of bone that project into each nasal cavity from the lateral side (Figure 1.7).

What happens while singing? The soft palate is elevated, blocking access of pharyngeal air vibrations to the nasopharynx and choanae. Nasal air vibration is therefore activated by sound vibrations transmitted by bone through the hard palate and the facial bones. When the size of the nasal cavities is compromised, such as by a deviated nasal septum or excessive reduction of the nose by overly ambitious rhinoplasty, nasal air vibration, proprioceptively perceived as the voice being "in the mask," is impaired. Conversely, when the nasal cavities are enlarged by straightening a deviated

THE VOCAL APPARATUS   17

septum and reducing the size of the turbinates, nasal resonance is increased. The voice is more easily "flipped up" into the mask, and the singer will perceive that the voice comes forward and may even sound louder. While nasal resonance is more important in terms of proprioception than acoustics, and not nearly as important as the pharynx in modifying the voice, it nonetheless plays a significant part in how the voice is perceived.

The final portion of the vocal tract is formed by the tongue, teeth, and lips. They play a minor role in shaping the voice, but a major one in articulating sounds and words, transforming vocal sound into speech and song. The tongue is the most mobile structure in articulation and functionally might be considered as playing two different roles (Figure 1.8). The posterior tongue (or attached tongue) is a shape-shifting mass of muscle that moves in basically four directions: up, down, backward, and forward. Depending on its position and shape, it can occlude or open the oropharyngeal resonating cavity. By moving up or backward toward the hard or soft palate, the posterior tongue also plays a role in articulating certain sounds (velar or palatal consonants).

The posterior tongue is connected below to the hyoid bone and, more anteriorly, to a flat muscular sheet (mylohyoid) that can also affect the position of the tongue: when the floor of the mouth is tensed, the tongue is pushed up into the mouth, and when relaxed, the tongue can drop and occupy less space intraorally. With excessive muscle tension the mylohyoid contracts and the tongue bulks up, reducing intraoral and oropharyngeal resonance. This results in a voice that is posterior and "covered." And here is another instance of how a singer must learn to deconstruct reflexive movements: when swallowing, the tongue and soft palate normally elevate at the same time, the tongue pushing the bolus of food back, and the palate rising to protect the nasopharynx. By contrast, singers need to separate these movements, lifting the palate while lowering the tongue, to increase the resonating space in the back of the throat.

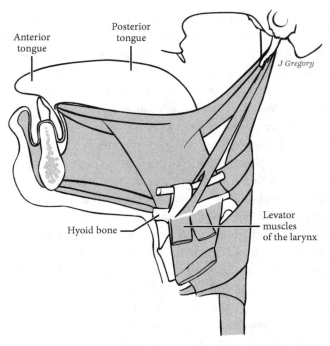

Figure 1.8 The anterior tongue is freely mobile. The posterior tongue rests on the floor of the mouth and is connected to the hyoid bone and, indirectly, to the larynx.

The anterior (free or unattached) part of the tongue is thinner and more versatile. This is the part that articulates words, particularly consonants. Unlike the posterior tongue, the tip has seemingly unlimited directional mobility and can normally touch any of the teeth, incisors to molars, as well as curl back to touch the soft palate. Its undersurface is partially connected to the anterior floor of the mouth by a thin band of fibrous tissue, the **lingual frenum**. If the frenum is abnormally short, it can have an adverse effect on tongue mobility and tension. We will discuss this condition, **ankyloglossia** or tongue tie, in greater detail later.

THE VOCAL APPARATUS   19

The importance of the tongue in voice production cannot be overemphasized. Its size, shape, length, mobility, and position in the upper vocal tract play a significant role not only in articulation but also in the location, magnitude, and harmonic spectrum of the voice that is produced.

Teeth, particularly the anterior upper teeth, are also involved in articulation, and sounds such as /d/, /n/, /t/, and /l/ are formed by placing the tip of the tongue against the back of the teeth or the alveolus, the ridge where the teeth are attached.

The lips play a role that is more complex. Anatomically, the lips form a sphincter, controlled by a ring of muscle, the **orbicularis oris.** The mouth can open or close, and the lips fully retract or pucker into whistle position, changing the acoustic characteristics of the oral cavity. Additionally, the lips are involved in determining the color of vowels and generate certain consonants (labial consonants), such as /p/. Since the lips form the final pathway where the voice leaves the body, they must be fully mobile with a good range of motion.

Although these parts of the vocal tract have less of a role in producing sound, they are extremely important, since sung words often need to be overarticulated to convey the textual information in a song or aria.

The Ultimate Resonator

When describing voice production, we usually forget the performance space. It is the ultimate resonator: the 500-lb. gorilla in the room **is** the room! The size and shape of the theater, the height of the ceiling, and the shape and the materials used to cover the walls and the floors all play a role in the listeners' auditory experience. Large performance spaces (such as cathedrals) with stone walls echo; small spaces may be too loud and "live."

20 KEEP YOUR SINGING VOICE HEALTHY!

As sound traverses the performance space, sound waves intersect, leaving specific spots that are acoustically responsive and others that are not. Where the singer is positioned on stage is also a factor, and experienced singers quickly learn where to stand for optimal sound.

2

From Function to Performance

The singing voice is the product of many elements, both structural and functional. The previous chapter covered some relevant aspects of the anatomy of the vocal apparatus and how they function to produce the voice. Now let's look more closely at how voice production becomes singing and correlate what happens functionally with what we hear.

Singing Naturally

By way of preamble, consider that the exhortation to "sing naturally" is deceptive. If "natural" means using the vocal tract as you find it, in its native state, then very few singers truly sing naturally. A choir of young untrained schoolchildren or perhaps villagers in a remote part of the world may be examples of truly natural singing.

By contrast, a trained singer, particularly in the classical genre, needs to use her vocal anatomy in a new and learned way that is often the opposite of how these structures naturally function. Table 2.1 lists some differences between the natural voice and the trained voice. Perhaps the instruction "to sing naturally" should be to "sound effortless"?

Table 2.1 contrasts the differences between singing with an untrained, "naïve" voice versus singing with a classically trained voice. We should qualify this comparison by saying that there are many other techniques employed by professional singers in nonclassical genres, such as jazz, pop, musical theater, and ethnic singing. These are often more effortful and involve a higher laryngeal position and

Keep Your Singing Voice Healthy! Anthony F. Jahn and Youngnan Jenny Cho, Oxford University Press.
© Oxford University Press 2024. DOI: 10.1093/9780197629703.003.0002

22 KEEP YOUR SINGING VOICE HEALTHY!

Table 2.1 Singing "Naturally" versus Trained Singing

Natural (Reflexive)	Artificial (Voluntary)
Laryngeal position high	Laryngeal position low
Pharynx moderately constricted	Pharynx open
Palate low	Palate raised
Vocal fold pressure: open or closed	Vocal fold pressure: moderated
No vibrato	Vibrato
Yodel	Passaggio
Normal inspiration/expiration ratio	Reversed inspiration/expiration ratio
Passive expiration	Active expiration
Thoracic breathing	Abdominal breathing
Mass reflexive movement of muscles	Individual controlled movement of muscles

more contracted pharynx. But the point we make is that any form of vocal training requires some modification, slight or substantial, of how the muscles involved in speech, respiration, and swallowing are used, a retraining that results in a voice that is certainly not "natural."

Vocal Registers and Transitions

A great deal of discussion and controversy have been generated by the topic of vocal registers. How many registers are there, and what are their defining characteristics? A detailed review of vocal registers is beyond the scope of this book. We will therefore simplify our discussion based on our understanding of laryngeal physiology.

The singing voice, from bottom to top, is divided into two main registers: **chest voice**, so named because the lower notes create a vibratory sensation in the chest, and **head voice**, felt in the skull and facial bones. Chest vibration occurs when the air spaces in the trachea and bronchi resonate with vocal sound. While these vibrations are not audible, they can be felt. Feeling for this resonance by placing the hand on the chest (called tactile fremitus) has been used by physicians in the past to localize chest disease. Vibrations in the face (or mask) are also tactile and sensed proprioceptively by the singer.

Based on our previous discussion of resonators, this distinction of chest or head voice makes sense. But the real difference lies in the vocal mechanism used to produce sound in these two registers. Figure 2.1 illustrates the different laryngeal muscles involved in chest voice and head voice.

To sing in chest voice, the vocal folds are approximated by the adductor muscles of the larynx, as well as the muscle of the vocal fold itself (vocalis, or thyroarytenoid). These are all muscles inside the larynx "box" and are attached to (or part of) the vocal fold. The adductors bring the vocal folds together, the unpaired interarytenoid muscle (in the back, between the two arytenoids) holds them in that position, and the vocalis muscle tightens and bulks up the vocal fold. The overall effect is to narrow the glottic opening and increase resistance against the exhaled airstream.

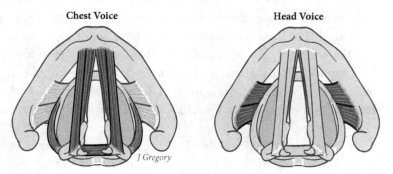

Figure 2.1 In chest voice, the vocalis, lateral cricoarytenoid, and interarytenoid muscles adduct the vocal folds. In head voice, the cricothyroid muscles contract and tilt the thyroid cartilage forward, elongating and further approximating the vocal folds.

The entire vocal fold vibrates in a wavelike fashion, the two folds oscillating symmetrically (Figure 1.3 in Chapter 1). As the pitch goes up, as with a slow *glissando*, the vocal folds continue to tighten, and their vibrating characteristics change.

At a certain pitch (usually around E ♭4 to F4 for sopranos), these "chest register" muscles are maximally contracted, and the upper limit of chest voice is reached. At this point, a register shift occurs, from chest to head voice. The adductors and vocalis muscles start to relax, and simultaneously, the cricothyroid muscles, attached to the outer surfaces of the thyroid and cricoid cartilage, contract, tilting the thyroid cartilage forward. The result? The vocal folds are passively stretched and indirectly approximated, becoming longer and thinner, and vibrating at a higher frequency.

As the pitch continues to rise, the cricothyroid muscles also reach their limit of contraction. Now, the vocalis muscle partially re-engages. This time, however, the effect is not so much to bulk up the vocal fold again (they've been stretched thin by the cricothyroid muscles) but rather to stiffen it. The surface membrane of the vocal fold, which initially vibrated as part of the entire fold, now decouples and, disengaged from the body of the vocal fold, vibrates independently. Video stroboscopic examination confirms that in this high range (usually above F5 for sopranos), only the very thin edge of the fold (i.e., the thin membrane covering the vocal fold) vibrates, while the body of the vocal fold is held stable between the combined pull of the vocalis muscle and the cricothyroid muscle. In men, this laryngeal posture produces a falsetto voice.

What we have described above corresponds to what happens as the voice goes from chest voice into high head voice. The cricothyroid muscle engagement represents the first transition (*primo passaggio*), and the decoupling of the superficial membrane represents the *secondo passaggio*. While both transitions result in a change in voice quality, the *primo passaggio* is more obvious: it involves a greater shift in terms of the laryngeal mechanism (and in what we hear), since it requires the simultaneous relaxation of one set of muscles and the contraction of another set.

Incidentally, these two different mechanisms also apply to the speaking voice, which can be produced in either chest or head register. The choice depends on many factors—cultural, habitual, and the desire to project a certain persona during speech.

Belting

The transition from chest voice into head voice may be compared to changing gears in a car with a manual transmission. In the hands of an experienced driver that shift can be smooth, while when driven by a student it can be jerky and rough. In vocal terms this translates into a gradual transition as one set of muscles relaxes and another set simultaneously engages.

Continuing the car analogy, there is an optimal engine speed where shifting can occur, or you might choose to rev the engine up more while staying in the lower gear and shift at a higher engine speed. In the same way, transitioning from chest into head voice can occur over a range of frequencies, although the optimal point becomes obvious with practice. Nonetheless, chest voice can be pushed higher, if the singer chooses, into what normally would be head range. The sound produced is more intense and urgent. Overuse of this technique (belting) may carry the same penalty as trying to drive your car faster while staying in second gear: it expends a lot of effort, uses a lot of gas, and may, over time, damage the engine. However, since belting is an important technique in popular genres, techniques for "safe belting" have been developed, which also engage the cricothyroid muscle, and so "blend" some head voice into the belt.

Vibrato

Vibrato, the rapid and periodic oscillation of the voice around a tonal center, is usually a learned technique. Historically, it has not always been part of the singer's bag of tricks. Certainly, straight tone singing, such as Gregorian chant or madrigals, and, more recently, ethnic singing, such as the villagers recorded by Bartok in the early 1900s (or the Bulgarian Women's choir), continue without the use of vibrato. In more popular genres such as jazz, vibrato is often added at the end of a longer tone, for color. In opera, however, most singing of longer notes uses this method.

Why vibrato? It is obviously a stylistic choice, and the type of vibrato used by singers has changed, as documented by early and more recent recordings. There are many other possible explanations, both technical and musical. Here are some possibilities. The rapidly alternating contraction and relaxation of vocal muscles allow the voice to sustain longer, by reducing the potential muscle fatigue induced by sustained contraction. By hovering around a tonal center (albeit in a controlled and regular fashion, as it pertains to both pitch fluctuations and periodicity), the task becomes more forgiving in terms of pitch accuracy, especially on longer tones. Through increasing the frequency of vibration, often along with a crescendo, the singer can impart a sense of growing urgency and importance to the melody. Musically, it may also have the effect of reinforcing the tone by repeated return to it from the minute and controlled excursions of pitch. Auditory fatigue (the decline in the alerting effect of a persistent straight tone) is overcome, and the listener's attention is focused on the forward impetus of vocal line. And finally, the inner ear is more effectively stimulated by this rapidly alternating sound. In this regard, it is interesting to consider that, when testing hearing in cases of severe hearing loss, audiologists have found that a "warble tone" is a more effective alerting stimulus for the ear, activating a broader group of hair cells in the cochlea.

Vocal Range

Vocal range refers to the series of notes, from bottom to top, that a singer can access. To be able to use the instrument well, a singer should ideally have at least two full octaves of usable notes, not counting a few additional notes on top that can be vocalized but not sung. That number is an approximation: most classical singers have more than two octaves, and there are many successful vocalists, usually in nonclassical genres, who have done well with a much smaller range. At the other extreme, Peruvian soprano Yma Sumac (1922–2008) was reputed to have a singing range of four and a half to five octaves.

Over a singer's working lifetime, vocal range is one of the more fluid assets: it can grow or decrease, but it is always changing. During school days, one of the young singer's goals is to discover her range, and the teacher's task is to guide this exploration, with the ultimate goal of fully accessing the entire voice, and, incidentally, uncovering the student's voice type. In the course of this journey, it may become apparent that a "mezzo" is really a soprano with a hitherto undiscovered upper range. Conversely, a "soprano" may discover her low notes and turn out to be a pants mezzo in the making. Singers with easy access to both high and low notes can decide which *fach* is more suitable, depending on voice quality and comfort.

As the singer passes the apex of her career, higher notes may become more difficult to access reliably. The power or color may change, or some notes become simply not comfortable and dependable. A change of *fach*, with corresponding change of repertoire, can sometimes accommodate this reality. Mezzos will often switch to lower roles, since chest voice usually continues to be strong. The degree and rate of this change vary depending on genes, technique, and repertoire choices. We will address the aging voice in more detail later, but the point here is simply this: the working vocal range of a singer is dynamic and not fixed, and impacted by many factors.

28   KEEP YOUR SINGING VOICE HEALTHY!

Voice Types

Voices may be high or low, and are usually divided into bass, baritone, and tenor for men, and alto, mezzo-soprano, and soprano for women. Where the voice lies, and especially where the voice sits most comfortably, is determined more by anatomy than physiology. The overall physique and facial structure can often give a clue to the voice we might expect to hear, and the vocal folds of a bass, thick, opaque, and often a little pinkish even at rest, are certainly different from those of a high soprano, whose vocal folds are thin, white, and at times almost bluish due to their translucency.

The subdivisions within these basic types, such as *basso profundo* versus *basso cantando*, or, among sopranos, the heavier *spinto* versus a lighter *soubrette* voice, pertain also to weight and color, and are more difficult to attribute to anatomy alone. Certainly, structural differences may play a role: two basses singing the same passage can sound quite different, one voice warmer and burnished, the other darker with a threatening, almost villainous, suggestion of a snarl. Each voice has its own inherent natural quality, and it would be difficult for one to convincingly mimic the other.

On the other hand, as the voice develops in a young adult singer, it often expands in range and even changes in *fach* without any obvious structural change. The determining factor here is function, as the singer is learning to use the same vocal apparatus in new ways. Finally, as the voice reaches maturity (and after maturity), it can change again, as a lyric soprano becomes more dramatic, or a lyric Mozart tenor moves into a heavier *verismo* repertoire. What is the determining factor here? This is more likely again due to structural changes, with function adapting to the structural reality of the older vocal apparatus.

Before leaving this topic, we should emphasize that the subdivision of voices by type (and *fach*), though useful, is somewhat arbitrary. Each voice is unique, and boxing them into a specific category is a bit like trying on a ready-made suit: the fit may not always be good. The same, of course, is true with repertoire. Unless you have had the good fortune of having a piece of music (or an opera) written specifically for your voice, you are faced with the task of wearing someone else's clothing, and the fit may be less than perfect.

The Speaking Voice

The speaking voice can also be centered in either the chest or head register. While singers spend years perfecting their singing voice, much less attention is given to speaking. This is regrettable, since even the most dedicated singer will spend most of her or his time speaking, using the same apparatus. The singing larynx is looked at almost as a separate structure, "the instrument," with every note carefully tuned, like a harp, and every phrase mindfully shaped. By contrast, the speaking voice is generally neglected: it is not an "instrument," but rather who we are! Whether we speak to teach, to convince someone, to tell jokes, or to complain, we don't pay attention to resonance or support: we're focused on the message. Since many singers support themselves through day jobs that often involve loud and constant speaking, we not uncommonly see patients with good singing technique who still develop vocal problems through faulty speaking habits. We have seen several Music Education graduates with good vocal training who after just one year of teaching in the public school system develop chronic muscle tension dysphonia, and even nodules.

How much of your vocal training can you carry over to your day job? While no one wants to carry on a conversation using a stagey voice, we recommend that you try to incorporate some singing technique into your speech. This is especially important if you are juggling your day job with a continued singing career. Take a big breath. You should speak with good support, and not on residual air. Since speaking in head voice involves less muscular

30   KEEP YOUR SINGING VOICE HEALTHY!

effort, women should consider speaking in head voice mix if that is comfortable. The frequency of your speaking voice should center around a comfortable range and should be continually modulated rather than monotonous. A modulated voice will hold the listener's attention with less laryngeal effort than a loud voice.

The speaking voice sends a message not only by content but also by pitch. Since speaking voice signals the persona you are trying to model, it is sometimes altered and becomes more effortful. At times, women executives in a male-dominated environment lower their voice to project more authority. Among male singers, we sometimes find that the speaking voice is altered to conform to the vocal *fach* the speaker is trying to project. Tenors may speak at a higher pitch than would be natural, and baritones who see themselves as basses may push their speaking pitch down and cover the voice to project the impression of a lower range.

In summary, the speaking voice need not always correspond to the singing voice (remember, some counter tenors are baritones), but it should be optimized, especially if you speak for a living. The best speaking voice is one that is the most comfortable to produce, and it is for this reason that we suggest you give your speaking voice as much thought as your singing voice.

3

Examining Your Instrument

A Hands-On Tour

Examining your larynx does not invariably mean a visit to the doctor. There is a great deal you can find on your own, just by palpating your own neck. We recommend this self-examination, since it not only provides familiarity and comfort but also can give some understanding of your normal baseline anatomy. We are often surprised at how little even some accomplished singers know about where the vocal folds are and in which direction they are oriented. So here is a quick guide to the normal surface anatomy of your vocal apparatus.

The purpose of this brief tour of the neck is to familiarize yourself with where these structures are and, in particular, with parts of the larynx that you can locate with your own hands. Be gentle, don't cause yourself discomfort, and don't be discouraged if you don't find everything: we are all different, and locating these surface landmarks in a long and thin neck is easier than in a shorter and thicker neck. However, if you do notice something that you can't identify, and particularly if it is only on one side or different on the two sides, you need to consult your doctor.

Begin in a comfortably seated position. Pointing your chin upward (Figure 3.1), you are now ready to explore the surface anatomy of your larynx. You can sit in front of a mirror, but your main focus should be on the sensation in your fingertips, since you will be palpating your neck manually. Using the point of your chin as a landmark, bring your fingers down the midline until you find your thyroid prominence. This prominence (formerly called the Adam's

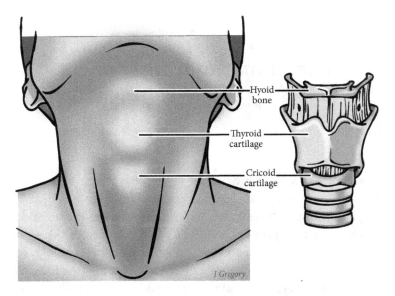

Figure 3.1 The surface contours of the anterior neck correspond to the anatomic features of the underlying larynx.

apple) corresponds to the V-shaped notch in middle of the top of the **thyroid cartilage.** It is easier to locate in men, since their thyroid cartilage is usually bigger and tilts forward. Placing your forefinger in the notch, you can now feel with your thumb and middle finger the upper margin of the thyroid cartilage forming the wings or flat plates of the cartilage on either side. You can gently run your fingers down the flat surface of each side of the cartilage. Unlike the soft cartilage of the ear or the nose, the two main cartilages of the larynx (thyroid and cricoid) are rigid and in later life may calcify and even partially turn into bone.

Now, place your thumb and forefinger back along the top edge of the thyroid. You will feel that they are actually in a groove. The lower edge of the groove is the upper rim of the thyroid. But the upper margin of the groove is formed by the **hyoid bone.** This small

EXAMINING YOUR INSTRUMENT   33

U-shaped bone is an important insertion point for several muscles that move the tongue, as well as muscles that raise the larynx. The gap between the hyoid bone and the thyroid cartilage (**thyrohyoid space**) may vary in width: it may be open and easily felt, or narrow and contracted. In classically trained singers who have learned to sing with a low larynx, this space is usually easy to find, whereas in non–classically trained or untrained singers, it can be quite narrow and barely discernible on palpation. If the area is tender, it is suggestive of excess muscle tension, excessive singing, or inefficient technique.

Palpating above the hyoid bone, in the area between the hyoid and the tip of the chin, you can feel some of the muscles that form the floor of the mouth and support the base of the tongue. As we start a swallow, these muscles contract reflexively and simultaneously: the tongue pushes back, and the larynx is raised and pulled forward. For effective singing, however, this area should normally be relaxed, soft and pliable, and not tense or tight. If these muscles are excessively contracted during singing, you may experience problems with tongue tension as well as a high larynx.

Let's return to the thyroid cartilage. Grasping the cartilage on either side, slide your thumb and forefinger down each side, until you feel a smaller firm circumferential prominence. This hard ridge is the **cricoid cartilage**, a ring of cartilage that forms the lower part of the larynx. Once you have located the cricoid, you can run your fingers along its surface to either side and feel it disappear under the muscles of the neck. It is a complete ring, round and prominent in the front and flattened in the back, an area where the arytenoid cartilages attach. You cannot feel this area. If you have sensitive fingers and favorable anatomy, however, you may be able to run your fingers on either side, along the **cricothyroid space**, a palpable groove between the thyroid (above) and the cricoid (below). If you do, you may notice that about halfway back, the groove disappears. This is the **cricothyroid joint**, where the thyroid cartilage is directly connected to the cricoid. It is here that the thyroid cartilage hinges, and, with contraction of the cricothyroid muscles, the thyroid cartilage tilts forward as the singer goes from chest to head voice.

Before we leave the larynx, grasp the thyroid cartilage again and, exerting a slight pressure toward the back of the neck, move it side to side. It should move relatively easily since it is attached only to muscles above and the flexible trachea below. You may feel a slight grinding or crunching sensation. This is normal! You are feeling the back of the cricoid cartilage rubbing against the neck vertebrae behind the pharynx, at the point where the esophagus begins. The two structures are separated only by thin layers of soft tissue, so this odd sensation, **laryngeal crepitance**, is normally present in most people.

You may wish now to examine the lateral parts of the neck. We suggest a gentle and limited exploration, to avoid pressing on the carotid arteries. You can gently look for the carotid arteries by feeling for the pulse in your neck, but avoid any pressure, since it may cause fainting. From the singer's perspective, you need only take note of two muscles in this area. The main strap muscles, beginning behind each ear and continuing down obliquely to the area where the top of the breastbone and the collar bone join, are the **sternomastoid** (sternocleidomastoid) muscles. These muscles are important in posturing and turning the head. They have no direct role to play in singing; however, excessive tightness or tension here can indirectly raise the tension in the laryngeal muscles. We will discuss this in greater detail in the chapter on laryngeal tension.

The second neck muscle you feel is the **trapezius**, a triangular-shaped muscle that forms the nape and connects the posterior neck to the shoulder. Once again, excess tightness in these muscles can have an adverse effect on voice production. Depending on your handedness or which side you carry your bag full of scores, one may be tighter than the other.

But what about the vocal folds? These, of course, are hidden, attached to the inside on the inside of the thyroid cartilage, about two-thirds down from the thyroid notch to the lower margin of the cartilage. They run back from that point (the anterior commissure) posteriorly to the arytenoid cartilages, which sit on top of the cricoid in the back. None of this can be palpated, but you may still be able to look at them yourself. How?

Many singers know that the vocal folds were first visualized not by a doctor but by a singer and voice teacher, Manuel Garcia (1805–1906). He used two handheld mirrors to reflect sunlight down into his throat in order to get a glimpse of his vocal folds. In an ingenious update on Garcia's technique, some singers have been using their mobile phones to look at their own larynx. We both have patients who do this routinely and who have gained some familiarity with what their own folds look like at rest and during phonation. While we don't advocate using this method to replace a medical examination or diagnosis, you might enjoy trying this for your own interest.

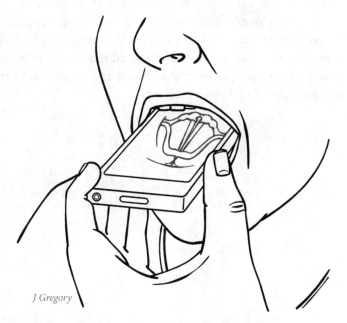

Figure 3.2 Visualizing your vocal folds using an iPhone.

36   KEEP YOUR SINGING VOICE HEALTHY!

If so, use a smaller mobile phone, since you will need to insert about half of it into your mouth. Clean the surface carefully, and then turn on the light on your phone. Insert the phone with the screen facing up and camera and light facing down (toward the tongue), in an oblique fashion, so the corner with the camera lens points to the back of your throat. Hold a hand mirror in your other hand to look at the image on the screen as you carefully advance the phone to the back of the pharynx. Try tilting the phone or changing your head position to make the image more apparent. You can now take pictures or make a video and, by using the mirror in your other hand, look at your larynx in real time. Please keep in mind, however, that you may not see the entire larynx in this way, since the anterior area may be hidden by the epiglottis. If you do see anything abnormal, however, and particularly if you are having vocal symptoms, you should see your doctor.

Depending on your curiosity and comfort level, we recommend that you familiarize yourself with your vocal apparatus. Although this does not replace a medical diagnosis, repeated self-examination may be reassuring and should reduce the anxiety of dealing with an instrument that is unseen and unknown. In this case, familiarity should breed comfort.

4

Monitoring Your Voice

While laryngologists may have some knowledge of the singing voice, we don't speak the same language as our patients. Our understanding comes mostly from what our patients tell us and from what we see on examination. Much of medicine is based on visual information, whether presented as X-rays, tests, photographs, videos, or even pathology slides. We unintentionally give preferential credence to things we see; in fact, there is almost an addiction to **seeing** results, whether reports, graphs, or images. Oddly, even with voice disorders, visual diagnosis has come to overshadow other methods of examination, such as touching or listening.

However, singers, who actually inhabit their voice (or, perhaps the other way, since their voice inhabits them!), have a completely different appreciation of their instrument. When we teach young doctors, we emphasize this simple maxim: **the diagnosis of voice disorders is primarily an auditory process.** This may seem obvious, but all of us, singers included, tend to be seduced by colorful images. Images are helpful but can also be distracting, even misleading. They certainly don't tell the whole story, and being told that "everything looks normal," when you know there is a vocal problem, is not reassuring, although unfortunately it is a frequent occurrence.

Singers experience their voice simultaneously in several ways, and none of them are visual. Hearing the voice is the most important. Sound travels to the ear by two paths, air conduction and bone conduction (Figure 4.1). **Air conduction** is hearing the voice as it comes out of the mouth, travels through the air, and enters the ears—normal hearing. **Bone conduction** refers to sound generated

Keep Your Singing Voice Healthy! Anthony F. Jahn and Youngnan Jenny Cho, Oxford University Press.
© Oxford University Press 2024. DOI: 10.1093/9780197629703.003.0004

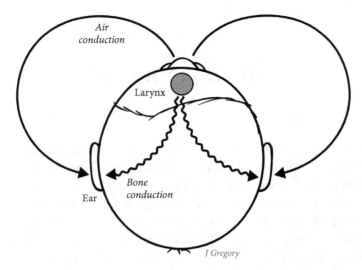

Figure 4.1 The voice travels to the ears by two pathways: through the air and through the bones of the skull.

inside the vocal tract that is transmitted directly through the skull to the inner ears. Like a vibrating tuning fork held to the head, the sound of our voice makes the facial and skull bones vibrate. Whether speaking or singing, we normally hear ourselves by both air and bone conduction.

But the two pathways don't transmit the same sound sensation. Since shorter sound waves don't propagate through bone as well as longer ones, bone conduction emphasizes lower sounds (like vowels), making the voice in our head sound richer but less distinct. Many of us who hear our recorded spoken voice for the first time are struck by the difference between what we hear as we speak versus what the recording tells us: the recorded sound is thinner and perhaps more nasal.

Voice monitoring by bone conduction can be useful or deceptive. It is useful—indeed, necessary—when singing with a loud orchestra or in ensemble singing. A choral singer's ear is overwhelmed by the voices around him, and internal sound monitoring becomes more important. On the other hand, when singing with congestion, the swollen mucous membranes in the vocal tract absorb more sound. Blocked ears may further decrease air-conducted hearing, and bone conduction becomes greater. This accounts for the mistaken notion of some people that their voice sounds better when they have a cold.

Singers also experience their voice physically, by **proprioception**. This third way is usually ignored by nonvocalists, but for singers a heightened awareness of feeling the voice is important, both during learning and by way of monitoring the voice during performance. Much of the imagery of vocal pedagogy hinges on "placing the voice," guided by proprioceptive appreciation of vocal vibrations. Depending on the register, the voice is felt in the chest, then in the head, specifically the facial area, or "mask." Our soprano patients tell us that as they access their higher notes, the voice seems to form a column and come out at the top of the head. Images such as voice placement, reflecting the voice off the palate, flipping the voice up into the mask, and bringing the voice forward all pertain to proprioception. The functional correlate of such imagery corresponds to areas of focal resonance in the upper vocal tract that are activated during voice production.

The last method for vocal monitoring is linked to **muscle memory**, or position sense. This is a problematic term, since it pertains not only to spindle receptors in the muscles that signal muscle position, tension, or relaxation but also to the brain's input. Position awareness is learned, but some position sense is innate. Some very young children can pitch-match without any vocal training. How does a singer find a particular note or negotiate a particular interval? It is certainly not by trial and error, like a beginning violin student who tries to find the right note on a string. When given a note and then asked to sing a major third above, the singer knows how to position the vocal folds, how to posture the resonators, how much air to exhale, and under how much pressure, even before that note is sounded. Further, she knows what to do to change the color of that note, all based on both innate ability and experiential learning. To attribute this to just "muscle memory" does not fully explain something that seems far more complex.

Tracking the voice in real time involves all four modalities working together. Air conduction hearing normally dominates, but any of the four may need to be called upon, depending on the singer's vocal health and performance circumstances. A good comparison is with a pilot who flies by a combination of vision and instrumental guidance. While hearing is the most accurate, none of the four is always completely reliable, and this may account for why even a capable singer may be sharp or flat: singing *fortissimo* in an operatic ensemble against a full orchestra may confuse the ear and leave the performer dependent on less exact modalities such as proprioception or muscle memory, rather than clearly hearing the pitch.

5

The Glissando Test

A Simple Vocal Checkup

How is your instrument today? Most experienced singers are viscerally familiar with their voice: they usually know every note, what it sounds like, how it feels, and what they need to do to sing today compared to yesterday. Much of this is proprioceptive, giving rise to the frequent, and medically puzzling, complaint of "the voice doesn't *feel* right," especially toward the top of the range.

Every singer has her own special tests to check the voice, so some of the suggestions here may therefore be unnecessary for you, but we offer a quick and easy way to check your voice that we have found useful, regardless of your voice type or singing genre.

You should know vocal range, bottom to top. How high can you sing, and how high can you vocalize? While trained singers can name their top notes, less experienced vocalists often cannot. We usually ask these questions and then independently confirm top and bottom, either using a keyboard or a keyboard app, such as Virtuoso. As mentioned earlier, we normally expect at least a two-octave working range. Since a common early sign of vocal trouble is difficulty with the highest notes, monitoring and documenting any changes here over time gives a good measure of any improvement or worsening. You can do this at home—no doctor's visit is necessary—but do it later in the day so the test is representative of your normal "warmed up" range, not your morning voice.

Keep Your Singing Voice Healthy! Anthony F. Jahn and Youngnan Jenny Cho, Oxford University Press.
© Oxford University Press 2024. DOI: 10.1093/9780197629703.003.0005

The Glissando Test

A few years , we developed the **glissando test** as a quick but informative voice check. This simple test gives a lot of diagnostic clues about your vocal health.

How is it done? You simply sing a very soft *glissando*, or "siren," sliding from the bottom to the top of your range, on an "eee" vowel (it is more difficult with open vowels and easier, but less diagnostic, sliding down). Try and do it on a single breath. Since it is hard to objectively listen while singing, we suggest that you record your voice and then listen to it critically.

Take a full breath, and then as softly as possible slide up, bottom to top—not a scale but a *glissando*. No *crescendo*, no *vibrato*—you're not performing but looking at the natural voice, warts and all. Sing softly, with a relaxed throat; avoid muscling or squeezing. You can make a couple of runs at it, although the first one is usually the most telling, before you figure out how to finesse the difficult spots. We don't want you to "get it right" but rather look more at why you may be getting it wrong.

And now you can put on your adjudicator's hat, push the playback button, and listen.

Listen first to the overall texture of the *glissando*: is it uniform or uneven in quality, with areas of strain? If the voice is hoarse throughout, there is obviously a problem. The commonest cause is laryngitis, and if you are also ill, coughing, and congested, general hoarseness is to be expected. There are of course other causes, but the main thing is to see whether over the next several days the hoarseness resolves on its own along with your other symptoms. If it persists, you should be evaluated.

Now focus on the transition from chest into head voice, the mix, or *primo passaggio*. Most beginners have a problem here just as a matter of inexperience, but even for trained singers this can be a difficult area to negotiate. A seamless transition from chest to head voice is usually the sign of a well-trained voice.

THE GLISSANDO TEST   43

For all singers, experienced or not, the *primo passaggio* is the most sensitive indicator of vocal tension. In fact, the first sign of muscle tension, even if mild, is usually a change in texture as the transition is negotiated. It may be just a momentary thinning of the voice, the fabric sounding a bit frayed, or an audible flip from chest to head register. Less often there is an actual gap, like a yodel. If you are technically at a stage where you normally have no difficulties here, any of the above changes are significant and should be noted.

A hole in the head voice, extending up from the *primo passaggio*, is another sign to be noted. As your *glissando* goes through this higher range, avoid a crescendo or increased muscling here, and the defect may become evident.

Next, listen to the voice around and above the *secondo passaggio*. Remember, this is where the body of the vocal fold (vocalis muscle and vocal ligament) tightens, and the surface membrane is set free to vibrate on its own. For this decoupling to take place, the surface membrane must be pliable and free of any swelling, and Reinke's space needs to be moist and slippery. Any difficulty around and especially above this transition is suggestive of swelling of the margin of the vocal fold. Depending on the degree of swelling, the hoarseness can be localized just to the region above the second passaggio (usually F5 and above) or can extend below it. While there is no direct correlation with the extent and depth of the swelling and the exact notes affected, it makes sense that if the surface membrane is swollen, it has greater mass than usual, and if the swelling extends deeper to interfere with decoupling at Reinke's space, the voice would be impaired. The range above the *second passaggio* may have become limited, and the sound might be breathy or even have a double pitch (diplophonia). All these abnormalities should be noted.

It is not uncommon to find that both transition points are impaired, especially if the voice has been hoarse for more than a day or two. The top may be hoarse, and there is also a defect in the *primo passaggio*. The two commonest reasons for this are either that vocal

44 KEEP YOUR SINGING VOICE HEALTHY!

fold swelling has led to increased muscling by way of compensation or (conversely) that persistent singing with muscle tension has caused excess trauma and swelling to the edge of the vocal folds. Muscle tension is an important topic, which we will discuss in a separate chapter.

While the **glissando test** is an excellent way to quickly check your voice for problems, we shouldn't overinterpret its diagnostic implications since it is difficult to definitively identify a problem without looking at the vocal folds. So, if you do hear anything abnormal, and especially if the problem persists despite voice rest or grows worse, a visit to the laryngologist is in order.

6

Hearing and Singing

Good hearing is important for good singing. It is the dominant part of the singer's feedback system: although singers monitor their voice in several ways, hearing your own voice, by both air and bone conduction, is the major guide.

How do we hear? The outer ears collect air vibrations in the environment. The sound waves travel along the ear canal to the ear drum (tympanic membrane), which is set into vibration. Attached to the inner surface of the ear drum is the first of a chain of three tiny bones. These bones, suspended in the middle ear, conduct the vibrations from the ear drum to the inner ear (cochlea). In the cochlea, mechanical vibrations generate an electric signal that the brain eventually perceives as "sound."

Normal hearing therefore involves two mechanisms, a **conductive** portion, which transmits mechanical air vibrations to the inner ear, and a **sensory** portion, which transforms vibrations to electric signals, beginning in the inner ear, and then transmitted through the auditory nerve to the brain. Impaired function in either mechanism can cause hearing loss. Some causes of conductive hearing loss may be blockage of the ear canal with wax, a hole in the ear drum, or fluid in the middle ear. Sensory loss may be caused by aging, noise trauma, or viruses. And if you happen to have both a conductive and a sensory problem (such as an older person with ear wax), you will experience hearing impairment from both, **mixed** hearing loss.

Figure 6.1 illustrates the anatomy of the ear. Sound travels through the outer ear and the ear canal, to the ear drum. The ear drum vibrates, and vibrations are transmitted through the

Keep Your Singing Voice Healthy! Anthony F. Jahn and Youngnan Jenny Cho, Oxford University Press. © Oxford University Press 2024. DOI: 10.1093/9780197629703.003.0006

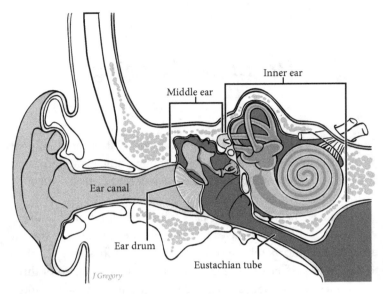

Figure 6.1 Cross-sectional diagram of the ear.

tiny bones of the middle ear to the inner ear, or cochlea. We normally hear sound through the ear canal, but sound waves can also set the skull bones directly into vibration. If you hold a vibrating tuning fork next to your ear, you hear the sound conventionally, through the air (**air conduction**). However, if you press the tuning fork against your head (behind the ear, or over the forehead), the vibrations bypass the outer and middle ear and travel directly through the skull bones to the inner ear (**bone conduction**). Like a tuning fork, your own voice is also partially absorbed into the skull and transmitted directly to the ears.

The singer's ear monitors the voice by both mechanisms. Air conduction picks up ambient sound as it comes out of the mouth and fills the air. Bone conduction picks up the vibrations absorbed by the walls of the vocal tract, which are transmitted through the skull to the inner ear. Both pathways are important, but both give slightly different information. Air-conducted sound, the sound in your

HEARING AND SINGING   47

environment, is high fidelity: you hear all the wavelengths present in the voice, along with the voices of the singers next to you, the orchestra or band, and environmental noise. Bone-conducted sound transmits your voice only, but it muffles the higher frequencies, so the lower frequencies dominate.

Hearing is the main mechanism for gauging the loudness and pitch of your voice, and if your hearing is impaired for certain frequencies, it is difficult to produce sounds in the range. An extreme example: when a severely deaf person speaks, the voice is soft and monotonous, and many of the high-frequency consonants are simply missing.

If significant hearing loss is **acute** in onset, the sudden change is readily perceived. A common cause is ear wax impaction or congestion affecting the middle ear, such as with a cold. These conditions cause **conductive** hearing loss, which is usually not serious. If hearing loss is due to an inner ear problem (**sensory** or nerve loss), however, it can be an emergency that requires medical treatment, so if you have a unilateral hearing loss, it is important to determine whether this is due to blockage (conductive loss) or an inner ear problem.

Is it conductive or sensory? Here is a simple test: close your mouth and hum loudly. You will hear the sound inside your head. Do you hear it more on the affected side or the normal side? If it is louder on the hearing-impaired side, you have a conductive hearing loss, which should be medically evaluated but can often be easily remedied. If, however, the sound goes to the "good" side, you may have nerve deafness. This is a potentially serious problem that requires urgent medical attention.

Acute (or sudden) hearing loss is usually obvious. More insidious is the **gradual** decrease in hearing, such as may occur with aging. This usually begins in the highest frequencies, well above the speech and singing range. As it worsens, the decrease in hearing first impairs high harmonics (such as those produced by an oboe) and then higher-frequency consonants, such as "s," "h," and "f."

Since the initial onset and rate of progression of age-related hearing loss vary, we suggest that every singer monitor their hearing after age 50, if only to get a baseline hearing test.

Two early signs of hearing loss are difficulty hearing in noisy environments and difficulty hearing the TV. For some reason, some accents are more problematic. To use our ears effectively in localizing a sound source, the hearing thresholds in the two ears must be within 10 decibels of each other, and a telltale sign of even a mild unilateral hearing loss is the inability to pinpoint where the sound is coming from.

Our ears are exquisitely sensitive to very soft levels of sound. They evolved at a time when there were no machines, sirens, or motorcycles and no loud music. In fact, our ears could not be more sensitive: it has been said that if they were, we would hear the molecules of our inner ear fluid bumping into each other (Brownian movement)!

Noise is the ubiquitous pollutant of our environment. It bombards us at a higher and more consistent level than our ears were designed for. Protecting the ears from noise (and loud music) is a lifelong task, and pop or rock singers are at greater risk for hearing loss. Singing with amplified accompaniment can cause gradual but irreversible damage to the ears. An early warning sign is temporary **tinnitus**, a ringing or hissing sound that persists for several hours after noise exposure. Over time, the damage caused by noise becomes permanent and, if it progresses, can eventually affect speech perception, necessitating the use of hearing aids. Noise-induced hearing loss is often accompanied by permanent tinnitus. For this reason, we recommend that you monitor the sound levels in your professional (and social) environment regularly.

How loud is too loud? Industrial (Occupational Safety and Health Association) standards recommend no more than 85 decibels sound exposure for an eight-hour workday. For shorter periods, such as a concert, the level of sound reaching your ears should be under 95 decibels. As sound levels increase, the amount

HEARING AND SINGING 49

of exposure that will cause permanent damage gets shorter and shorter. Exposure to sound levels of 110 decibels for only one minute can cause permanent hearing loss. To monitor your noise exposure, we recommend that you download one of several free sound level meter apps available for your cell phone. This will prevent inadvertent exposure to damaging ambient noise, whether in a bar or at a concert.

Although you may not be able to always control the sound environment, you can reduce noise damage with the use of custom-fitted "**musicians' ear plugs**." While normal ear plugs reduce higher frequencies disproportionately, these high-fidelity plugs reduce all frequencies to the same degree (either by 15 or by 25 decibels), allowing you to appreciate the ambient sound spectrum in its normal proportions while preserving your hearing. Even when not performing, singers may find themselves in a social environment that is excessively noisy and potentially damaging.

An important consideration when using your voice in a noisy environment is the **Lombard effect**. This is an involuntary reflex whereby we inadvertently raise our voice when speaking over background noise. In effect, your brain tells you to raise your vocal volume to about 35 decibels above ambient sound, so that you may be heard. Put in practical terms, if you are in a normally quiet room (background noise under 50 decibels), you will speak at 85 decibels. However, on a noisy street or socializing in a busy restaurant or bar, where the ambient sound level is 80 or 90 decibels, you can unwittingly put out 120 decibels of vocal sound. Now, if you're yelling over background music or other people, perhaps disinhibited by alcohol, you may well go even louder than that. The effect on your larynx is increased muscle tension and possible vocal fold trauma. In a different setting, this phenomenon also affects choral singers, who need to guard against oversinging.

Can you still sing if you have impaired hearing? Of course you can. Many rock singers continue to perform well, despite significant noise-induced hearing loss and tinnitus, even though in daily

50 KEEP YOUR SINGING VOICE HEALTHY!

life their hearing loss poses an increasing handicap. Over the years we have also seen several prominent classical performers who sing with hearing aids. However, this is a new learning curve, since the sound of a hearing aid is quite different from normal hearing, and hearing-impaired singers need to reinterpret the sound they produce, as well as rely more on nonauditory (propriocep-tive) monitoring of their voices. It is a functional but suboptimal second choice: better to preserve your hearing while young than attempting to remedy an important sense organ once it becomes damaged.

7

Muscle Tension and the Voice

Excessive muscle tension is a common problem for many singers. We instinctively know how to *contract* muscles: it is an active process, and how every part of our body moves. How to *relax* muscles, however, normally does not attract our attention, and awareness needs to be learned. While "active relaxation" sounds like an oxymoron, it is in fact an important skill for singers: learning how to contract specific muscles, or muscle groups, while simultaneously relaxing others.

Most muscles that are potentially under voluntary control (called **striated muscles**, and different from involuntary **smooth muscles**, such as those that cause intestinal contraction) are arranged in opposing agonist-antagonist pairs. To work optimally, one muscle contracts while its opposite relaxes. The principle is the same whether we think of the biceps and triceps of the upper arm, the muscles that raise and lower the larynx, or the muscles that open and close the vocal folds.

If we include stance, support, and neck-torso alignment, we could say that singing involves almost every muscle of the body. However, singing primarily activates the muscles of the chest, abdomen, and vocal tract. Breathing and vocal fold movement use muscle activity that can work either reflexively or voluntarily: we can cough or take a deep breath, either automatically or on purpose.

In addition to "active relaxation," a key task for singers is to gain conscious and selective control over individual muscles that normally contract subconsciously and *en masse*. This requires deconstructing involuntary reflexive sequences, such as those involved in breathing or swallowing, into its discrete elements, first

Keep Your Singing Voice Healthy! Anthony F. Jahn and Youngnan Jenny Cho, Oxford University Press.
© Oxford University Press 2024. DOI: 10.1093/9780197629703.003.0007

gaining proprioceptive awareness, and then developing voluntary control of its individual muscular components.

The best example of this is how singers lower the larynx. For the untrained, this would also involve the tongue and the hyoid complex, all contracting and pushing back together. Singers, however, need to learn how to contract the depressor muscles of the larynx in isolation. The effect, lowering the larynx while keeping the muscles of the tongue and floor of the mouth relaxed and in their normal position, enlarges and elongates the hypopharyngeal resonant cavity, resulting in a voice that is bigger and richer. This posture is not natural and must be learned. Like most skills, once consciously learned, it becomes subconscious and "normal."

What happens when opposing groups of muscles contract simultaneously? Like a tug of war, it depends on the strength of the team pulling on either side. If the agonist-antagonist muscles are matched in strength and number and they pull equally hard, the result is no net movement (isometric contraction). By way of example, if we lock our fingers and try to pull our arms apart, both arms are equally strong, and the hands don't move.

But this is not what happens with the larynx. As mentioned earlier, since protection of the airway during swallowing is the highest priority, the muscles raising the larynx are greater in both number and strength than the depressors that pull the larynx down Figure 7.1). Similarly, the muscles that approximate the vocal folds (adductors) are both stronger and more numerous than those that abduct them. In fact, there is only one paired abductor (the posterior cricoarytenoid), whereas there are three paired adductors (the lateral cricoarytenoid, the thyroarytenoid, and the much more substantial cricothyroid), as well as the unpaired interarytenoid.

So what happens if all these muscles were to contract equally and simultaneously (isotonic contraction)? The stronger team wins, with the net result that the vocal folds would tightly approximate (adductors overpower the abductor) and the larynx would rise up to a higher position in the neck (elevators beat depressors). And

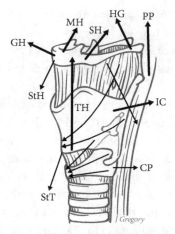

Figure 7.1 Diagram showing the direction of pull of the muscles responsible for raising or lowering the larynx. The elevators far exceed the depressors, both in number and in force.

PP, palatopharyngeus; HG, hyoglossus; SH, stylohyoid; MH, mylohyoid; GH, geniohyoid; StH, sternohyoid; TH, thyrohyoid; IC, inferior constrictor; StT, sternothyroid; CP, cricopharyngeus. (Modified from Sir Victor Negus: The Mechanism of the Larynx, 1929.)

this is just what happens, to varying degrees, when singing with excessive muscle tension.

Excessive muscle tension impairs the singing voice in several ways. Since the folds are approximated primarily by rotating the arytenoids inward, what happens when they are overrotated? The tips of the cartilage (vocal process) in the back of the vocal fold push against each other so hard that a gap opens behind them. This posterior gap creates an escape for air that normally drives the vocal folds, resulting in a breathy sound and decreased vocal power. Since the vocalis muscles remain tight throughout phonation, they resist the elongating effect of the cricothyroid, and head voice becomes effortful and limited.

The walls of the larynx above the folds (the supraglottic larynx) and the pharynx also contract, including the false vocal folds. The space above the vocal folds narrows. The ventricles (the small niches between the true and false vocal folds) are squeezed shut. This is the resonator that normally activates the "singer's formant," a high overtone that allows the voice to ring and soar above the orchestra.

In effect, the entire pharyngeal resonator is made smaller: bottom to top (the larynx is pulled up) and in circumference (the walls are pulled in). As the muscular walls of the resonator are "flexed," they become firmer, less absorptive, and more reflective. The result is a voice that is smaller, lacking in color and projection, and demonstrating a harsher, metallic quality, which may be accompanied by the physical discomfort of excessive muscle effort.

Muscle tension dysphonia (MTD) can occur for many reasons, some intrinsic to the larynx (primary), but many more due to extrinsic causes that are not directly caused by phonation (secondary). Primary MTD, the use of excessive or incorrect muscular effort in phonation, is most often found in beginners who have not yet learned to properly manage the selective contraction and relaxation of the muscles of the vocal tract. The untrained singer often has a high larynx, singing with great effort and, sooner or later, discomfort. For singers early in their training it is a significant discovery that, contrary to expectations, the more you push and squeeze, the smaller the voice becomes. No surprise here, considering that most of the amplification occurs in the pharynx, and increased muscle tension diminishes the size of this resonator. Other causes of primary laryngeal tension include injudicious belting, unsupported singing, which is sometimes seen in more popular genres such as rock; and singing excessively, especially a new or more strenuous repertoire. In such cases, MTD can occur even in trained singers.

Implicit in our discussion of "vocal training" is the assumption that singers are trained in Western classical technique. There are, however, many parts of the world where "classical" singing involves a high larynx, a tight pharynx, and a muscled sound. Folk music or pop music in India or the Arab countries, for example, uses this

MUSCLE TENSION AND THE VOICE   55

technique, and singers we have examined from these parts of the world often demonstrate signs of what we in the West would consider excessive muscle effort.

The Tongue and Tongue Tension

Overcoming **tongue tension** is a major hurdle for many singers. The tongue is a highly mobile structure made up of muscle tissue and is the strongest muscle within the vocal tract.

In terms of function, the tongue has two parts, mobile and fixed. The anterior portion is thin and moves freely in multiple directions. It is involved in speech as well as in tasting and manipulating food, and usually moves in a selective and consciously initiated manner. The posterior tongue is thicker and attached to the floor of the mouth. It moves up and down, bulking up to push food to the molars on either side, and then pushing the chewed-up bolus backward to initiate the swallow. The posterior tongue muscles connect to the floor of the mouth and the hyoid bone, which also provides attachment to the levator muscles of the larynx. Movements of the posterior tongue are more reflexive but, like other parts of the vocal tract, can be voluntarily initiated and controlled.

The tongue plays a major role in singing. The anterior tongue is involved in articulation of the text. Proper pronunciation of consonants requires the tongue to move freely in relationship to the teeth and palate, and these movements are coordinated with movements of the lips and the jaw. Dental consonants (such as "d" and "t") involve the tongue tip, while velar consonants (such as "k" and "g") require approximating the tongue with the palate. Since singers must learn to overarticulate for the sake of clarity, free mobility of the anterior tongue is important.

The main vocal effect of the posterior tongue consists of modifying the resonating space in the back of the throat by virtue of its shape and position. When the posterior tongue bulks up, oral and oropharyngeal resonance is reduced. If the posterior tongue is pushed back, it occludes the oropharynx, creating a "covered voice." A covered voice is darker and emphasizes the lower frequencies. It can be used as a special effect, although some, especially lower male voices, use this more routinely to create the impression of a lower range. In inadequately trained singers, a pushed-back tongue may be part of an attempt to lower the larynx.

By its attachment to the hyoid, the tongue is connected to other muscular structures in the upper airway, and a tense tongue goes hand in hand with tension in the floor of the mouth, pharynx, and larynx. Under typical circumstances, learning to relax the tongue (and floor of the mouth) is just a part of deconstructing the reflexive mass movements engaged by breathing and swallowing. When we examine the mouths of trained singers, one clue to good tongue control is that they can flatten the tongue voluntarily. Untrained patients usually hump up the back of the tongue as they open the mouth, whereas in trained singers the tongue forms a concave trough, hugging the floor of the mouth.

Tongue Tie and Muscle Tension

Some singers continue to struggle with tongue tension well into their career. While this may be just a persistent technical problem, in several cases we have identified an anatomic cause, which is potentially treatable. We are referring to **ankyloglossia**, or tongue tie.

The undersurface of the anterior tongue is connected to the floor of the mouth by a thin band of tissue, the lingual frenum. In most cases the frenum is of adequate length and allows the tongue to move freely. When the frenum is of long enough, you should be able to touch the tip of the tongue to the upper frontal incisors with the mouth fully opened. However, when it is too short, it anchors the tongue (ankyloglossia), limiting its movements. The frenum in such cases acts as a restraining tether, and the tongue is

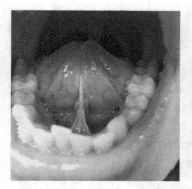 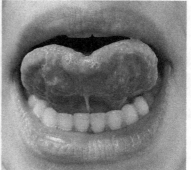

Figure 7.2 Two examples of severe anterior tongue tie. Note how the short frenum limits both the upward lift and the protrusion of the tongue.

left straining against its "leash," raising general lingual muscle tension (Fig 7.2).

There are many adults with a short lingual frenum, and usually they have learned to compensate. For nonsingers, the issue is primarily learning how to produce dental and alveolar consonants, and they do this by not fully opening the mouth during speech. However, this also increases muscle tension in the jaw, so it is not an optimal solution for singers. Having said that, not every singer with tongue tension has a tongue tie, and, conversely, not every singer with even moderate degrees of tongue tethering is affected.

But there is more. The tongue can be tethered in more than one way. The visibly short and taut lingual frenum forms an anterior tongue tie, restraining the tongue tip. However, in some cases the fibers also occur deeper, within the substance of the tongue, tethering the tongue posteriorly. Now the midportion of the tongue is also limited in range of motion, affecting velar consonant articulation, and further heightening the resting muscle tension in the tongue. A telltale sign of a posterior tongue tie is a visible dimple when the tongue is fully extended.

Case Report

A 32-year-old soprano presented with persistent vocal difficulties in the transition from chest to head voice (primo passaggio). Despite this problem, she has had a successful international career, but tension in the middle voice has always been a problem for her. She also admitted to chronic tongue tension, which she has been unable to overcome despite years of assiduous effort.

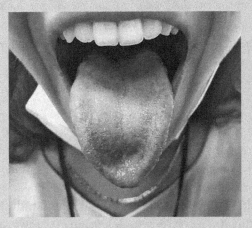

Figure 7.3 Posterior tongue tie. A fibrous band within the muscle tethers the tongue, causing the appearance of a dimple.

Examination confirmed signs of laryngeal muscle tension. Significantly, on extending her tongue, a midline dimple was seen due to tethering by a posterior tongue tie (Fig 7.3). This had not been previously noted. She was advised to consider having the condition treated.

Comment

Although even moderate limitations in tongue movement can be overcome by compensatory posturing, the effects of heightened muscle tension in the tongue persist and can have a negative impact on singing.

If the tongue is tethered, this can impair articulation of consonants, but the effect depends on which part of the tongue needs to move to produce certain sounds. And since the articulation of some consonants varies in different languages, the problem can be very specific: one of our patients complaining of muscle tension dysphonia told us that he was changing his repertoire from German to Italian. He had an anterior tongue tie, which caused no problems when singing a German "r" sound (posterior) but caused tongue tension when singing an Italian "r," which involves the tongue tip.

This is new knowledge: we have only recently begun to appreciate the link between tongue tie and tongue tension. It is an important finding for several reasons. It represents an anatomic cause for tongue tension, which may be corrected. But the more general issue is its effect on raising muscle tension elsewhere in the vocal mechanism. Since the tongue works in concert with the jaw, jaw tension, along with increased tension in other muscles of speech and singing, may develop and persist unless the cause is identified and corrected.

Garden variety tongue tension can often be greatly improved by massaging the tongue and the floor of the mouth. Here is a simple routine we recommend, which can be implemented daily if necessary and takes only a few minutes.

Sit comfortably, with good posture. Relax your jaw into a slightly open position. Move your tongue, pointing the tip in four directions, like stretching your muscles before exercise. If tongue elevation is limited, slide both thumbs into the mouth and under the tongue, and gently push up. The key is gentle but persistent pressure.

Using the thumb and forefinger, gently pinch the upper neck, just under the chin. Now massage the area between the chin and the hyoid bone. Stay away from the lateral parts of the neck. Slide your fingers down the neck on both sides, moving the hyoid and the larynx toward the top of the sternum. Most tongue-related tension

60   KEEP YOUR SINGING VOICE HEALTHY!

is concentrated in this part of the neck, but gently pulling the top of the thyroid cartilage downward also lowers the larynx and releases tension between the hypoid and the thyroid.

If despite careful practice and massage you have persistent muscle tension in the tongue and anterior floor of the mouth, consider the possibility of a hitherto overlooked tongue tie. If this is your problem, myofunctional therapy or minor surgery may release your tongue, with positive consequences.

Jaw Tension: The Daily Grind

The strongest muscles in the head are the two **masseter** muscles, which close the jaw. When we bite down, our molars can exert a force of 162 lbs. per square inch. Since the muscles that are involved in singing need to open the jaw and move it freely to articulate words, unintended masseter muscle tension may be a potential impediment.

The mandible, or lower jaw, is hinged on both sides in front of the ear, forming the temporomandibular joint, or TMJ. The joint consists of a ball-shaped head on the jaw, which swivels and slides against the side of the skull, as the mouth opens and closes (swiveling) and we chew with our molars (sliding). The movements also correspond with the abnormal habits of clenching and grinding. You can feel the TMJ in front of your ears, and even better by placing your little fingers, facing forward, in both ear canals while opening and closing the mouth.

When we eat, the jaw and tongue work together. We begin by biting the food with our incisors, the jaw opening and closing like a hinge. We then move the food backward onto the top of the tongue. The tongue humps up, pushing the food to either side, to the molars, which grind up the food (the jaw now in a sliding motion). The ground-up food is then pushed back toward the middle by the cheek muscles. The tongue now acts like a piston and pushes the food backward, to begin the oral phase of swallowing. The jaw, teeth, cheeks, and tongue work together smoothly, in a reflexive sequence. Since the main function of the jaw is chewing and clenching the teeth against resistance, the closing muscles are far stronger than those that open the mouth. While the muscles involved in chewing and grinding are different (clenching with the *masseter* and grinding with the *pterygoid* muscles), the effect on the jaw, teeth, and TMJs is similar. Under normal circumstances the food should be distributed to molars on both sides, and the pressure of the bite and the grind is exerted equally on both TMJs.

However, it turns out that most of us have a favorite chewing side! This is by habit, and normally we don't even think about it. It may have started years ago, perhaps with a sore tooth on the other side. It could also have begun after dental work, if the occlusion has changed or become uneven or a filling on one side was left too high. In any case, when the work of "food processing" is asymmetrically distributed, the pressure transmitted to the TMJs is unequal.

Chewing is normally intermittent, and the jaw muscles have some time to relax between meals, although some people habitually hold their jaw in a tensed position, unable to allow the muscles to fully relax. Clenching and grinding, known as **bruxism**, causes persistent tension in the jaw muscles as well as strain on the TMJ. There are numerous causes of bruxism. Some, such as allergic itching in the back of the throat, are treatable. In many cases, however, it reflects stress and tension: you grit your teeth in the face of adversity! Clenching often occurs at night while we sleep, and the only symptom is a sore jaw or earache on awakening (as well as possible complaints from your bed partner!). Persistent bruxism, in addition to heightening muscle tension in the jaws, can result in abnormal wear patterns on the teeth, as well as inflammation (and eventual damage) to the TMJs.

As with the muscles that lift and lower the larynx, the muscles that open and close the jaw are also unequal in both number and

62 KEEP YOUR SINGING VOICE HEALTHY!

strength: the closers (the temporalis, but mainly the masseter) are much stronger than the openers. So, if general muscle tone is raised, the result is a jaw that becomes more difficult to open and move side to side. From the singer's point of view, chronic tension in the jaw muscles limits opening the mouth during singing. In addition to possibly decreasing the volume of sound, it can also change the quality of the voice, since the resonant qualities of the oral cavity for vowels are subtly altered.

Further, clenching increases tension in adjacent muscles in the neck and the larynx. As mentioned earlier, generally increased muscle tension raises the larynx, constricting the hypopharyngeal resonating space. This not only decreases vocal power and resonance but also can lead to increased muscling, as the singer tries to compensate. In addition to muscle tension, which causes discomfort on opening and closing the jaw and even tenderness over the sides of the head, chronic bruxism can, over time, damage the TMJs.

There are a couple of ways that you can check whether you have the habit of clenching or grinding. If you wake up with jaw tension or feel discomfort in front of the ears, you should suspect bruxism. Put your fingers over these areas and open your mouth. If you feel tenderness over the joint, you have a problem. If you can feel a click or grinding on either side, this is a sign of structural damage to the joint. Another telltale sign is evidence of abnormal wear on the teeth. Since bruxism involves tooth-to-tooth pressure and contact, there may be visible changes involving the size, shape, and even color of the teeth.

For a simple and quick check, open your mouth and look at your upper front teeth. Your frontal incisors are normally shaped like a rectangle, with rounded "shoulders" at the corners. When the teeth are damaged by bruxism, the occlusal surface is ground down; the gently curved shoulders are truncated, leaving sharp corners; and the normally smooth horizontal cutting edges of the teeth may be chipped or irregular (Fig. 7.4).

MUSCLE TENSION AND THE VOICE   63

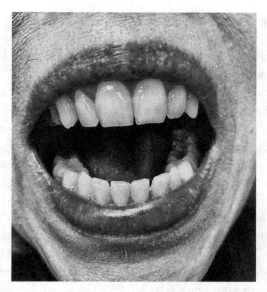

Figure 7.4 An avid amateur singer with a history of bruxism. Although the problem is now controlled with a nighttime oral appliance, previous clenching and grinding has left its mark on both upper and lower teeth.

There are many ways to manage jaw tension. First, some common-sense steps: have your dentist check your teeth for any abnormal wear. These include changes in the shapes of the incisors, canines, or molars, depending on whether the force of bruxism is exerted in the front or the back. Next, analyze your chewing behavior. When you eat, try to consciously chew your food on both sides. When eating something firm, like apples, "preprocess" your food in the front, since the farther back you chew, the more the jaw needs to open, putting the muscles at a mechanical disadvantage and straining the TMJ. Take smaller bites and precut that big apple before eating.

Avoiding chewing gum is common sense. If you feel tension, drop the jaw (like you learn to do when beginning voice lessons), letting it go slack. Also move the jaw side to side with the mouth open, to stretch and relax the muscles. Active and selective relaxation, a basic skill in effective singing, is nowhere more important than when dealing with the masseter.

Like many functional disorders, bruxism is often the result of other issues, and management of jaw tension can be complex, involving muscle relaxants, biofeedback, Botox, and even psychotherapy. But even if you don't experience any obvious signs of jaw tension, such as sore jaws in the morning, pain or tenderness over the TMJs, or limitation of mouth opening, you should consider lesser degrees of jaw tension as a possible culprit when it comes to muscle tension affecting your singing.

If you think you are experiencing symptoms of chronic jaw tension, here is a simple do-it-yourself routine to obtain relief. Once an hour, curl up your tongue and touch the roof of your mouth. This slackens your jaw slightly. Take a slow deep breath through your nose, and exhale through your mouth. At the same time gently massage both sides of your jaw (masseter) and temple (temporalis). This will draw your attention to these areas, remind you to relax the muscles, and break the unconscious clenching habit. Do this for one minute and repeat every hour.

We would like to offer a final word about oral appliances. These are devices that protect the teeth at night to reduce clenching and grinding. Their main benefit is to prevent tooth damage, by preventing your teeth (upper and lower) from gnashing against one another. Appliances can also change the jaw position and can reduce the force of the clench. They do not, however, stop clenching and grinding, and we have seen many patients who, over time, have chewed through their oral appliances. The other problem, with appliances that move the lower jaw forward to reduce snoring, is the increased strain on the TMJ caused by this displacement. So, while such oral appliances help, they are not the cure-all, and certainly do not fully eliminate the vocal consequences of increased muscle tension in the jaw.

Compensation-Related Muscle Tension

Laryngeal tension may also arise from persistent compensatory mechanisms developed to overcome a vocal impairment. For example, when dealing with transient vocal fold swellings, many singers muscle the voice to approximate the folds more forcefully. Of course, the voice will not be normal, but it will be adequate to get through the performance. Once the original problem resolves, however, it is important to undo this compensatory behavior and return to good normal vocal technique. If the singer has no conscious awareness that muscling has developed, it may persist, and now the compensation becomes the disease.

Longer-term vocal tension can occur in older people, where the vocal folds have atrophied (lost muscle substance) and can no longer adequately approximate with normal adduction. These patients have learned to engage excessive muscle force to squeeze the folds together. This creates other problems also, but with this extra muscle effort the voice becomes more audible.

Repertoire and Muscle Tension

Muscle tension dysphonia most commonly results from excessive vocal effort. This, in turn, may be in response to the demands made on the vocal apparatus, even in the absence of any other muscle tension in the body. Obvious causes, such as inadequate technical training or crossing over into a genre that requires more muscular effort, have already been mentioned. We need, however, to consider a few problems that are specific to opera singers.

Regardless of training, experience, or effort, there is a finite physical limit to how loud an unamplified singer can sound. If the theater is too big or the acoustics not supportive, the opera long and the on-stage time excessive, the voice may tire. It takes less vocal effort to fill a smaller theater, or one where the acoustics are

KEEP YOUR SINGING VOICE HEALTHY!

better. In 1805, when Beethoven's opera *Fidelio* was premiered, the Theater an der Wien was the biggest opera house in Vienna, with a seating capacity of almost 2,000. Today, the same work is sung at the Metropolitan Opera House, with a seating capacity of almost 4,000. The theater is twice as big, but the size of the soprano's larynx has not changed. And while many singers are (wonderfully!) up to that task, there are many others with beautiful voices who are not.

In the competitive world of opera, young singers are at times enticed or coerced into singing larger roles than they are capable of. The voice may not be ready for that role yet, but the opportunity is difficult to pass up. Perceived career advancement and financial considerations are other factors, supported by the conductor's promise (not always kept) that he will "keep the orchestra down." Once on stage, the demands on the larynx prove excessive. While many singers' voices mature over the years and eventually are capable of these larger roles, there are others whose voices, while beautiful, are simply not, regardless of age or experience. And once that transition to what may be an inappropriate repertoire is made, it is difficult to turn back. The signs of vocal burnout, such as a wide wobble, set in, and the career ends prematurely. One of an internationally known tenor's colleagues told us that excessive and overly effortful singing over the years affected his voice to the point where he became dependent on routine and frequent cortisone injections just to be able to sing.

Secondary Muscle Tension

Secondary laryngeal tension occurs when an unrelated condition triggers reflexive contraction of laryngeal and pharyngeal muscles. A common cause is **acid reflux**. If gastric acid refluxes into the pharynx, it causes inflammation of the mucous membranes and irritation of the underlying muscles. The muscles may then develop a higher resting tone, remaining in a state of partial contraction.

MUSCLE TENSION AND THE VOICE 67

The net result is a tight throat and an elevated larynx, which affect phonation.

Another example is "**laryngitis**" that develops with a sore throat. These patients usually have a pharyngeal infection with pain, or discomfort on swallowing, and then lose their voice. When we examine the larynx, however, we often find, to our surprise, that the vocal folds are rather normal in color, with only minimal swelling, and certainly not enough to account for a complete loss of voice. What happens, we believe, is that inflammation irritates the underlying pharyngeal muscles, causing them to contract. This raises the larynx to a degree that phonation becomes difficult. By massaging the muscles and releasing the larynx, the voice can often be restored in these patients within a few minutes.

An interesting example of excessive laryngeal tension is when a patient loses her voice for no apparent reason. There are usually underlying psychological issues at work here, such as somaticizing stress or secondary gain. On examination, the vocal folds are involuntarily held apart, in a position where no sound can be produced. Such posturing abnormalities need to be addressed with understanding and therapy, not with medication.

Case Report

A 35-year-old woman presented with a complaint of complete loss of voice. She could only communicate in whispers. She was otherwise well, with no evidence of infection or other symptoms. Examination revealed that her vocal folds were held apart and she was unable to approximate them to make a sound. On further questioning, she told us that, as a secretary, she had worked for years for an abusive boss who was constantly bullying and scolding her. One day, he yelled at her: "You are so stupid, it would be better if you said nothing at all!" The next day, she lost her voice.

68 KEEP YOUR SINGING VOICE HEALTHY!

> **Comment**
> This is a classic case of functional (formerly hysterical) aphonia. While we were able to restore her voice by manipulating the larynx, long-term management obviously required dealing with the intolerable psychological stress of her work environment.

Regardless of the cause, laryngeal tension can be confirmed by palpating the thyrohyoid space. Typically, this groove between the thyroid cartilage and the hyoid bone becomes narrowed or seems to disappear as we feel for it. The area can also be tender, a finding more common in cases where laryngeal tension is due to vocal misuse. Palpating the neck above the hyoid may also demonstrate tightness in the muscles of the floor of the mouth.

Muscles are always active, even when relaxed. This activity, the **resting tone of the muscle**, can be seen demonstrated using electromyography electrodes: even fully at rest, the muscle tissue demonstrates a few spikes of electric activity. Learning to "actively relax" means reducing this activity, the resting tone, to its lowest level. Stress or incomplete relaxation can raise the resting tone in any part of the body, a situation that is not helpful if we wish to function optimally.

In the vocal tract, irritation of the muscles, as in a pharyngeal infection or gastric reflux, has this effect. Interestingly, however, even muscles that are at a great distance from the larynx can increase laryngeal tension. This phenomenon, called **reinforcement**, can account for cases of laryngeal tension even in well-trained singers, where there is no apparent cause.

How does reinforcement work? Medical students are taught to check their patients' deep tendon reflexes by tapping the knee just below the kneecap with a small rubber hammer. The resulting knee jerk can be minimal or sizeable, depending on the resting tone of the muscle, but the amplitude of this reflex can be greatly increased simply by tensing muscles elsewhere in the body. For example, if the patient clenches his jaw tightly or interlocks his fingers and tries to pull the hands apart during the test, the knee-jerk reflex is dramatically enhanced: **increasing muscle tone or contraction anywhere in the body will raise the resting muscle tone in every other muscle!**

How does this apply to singing? It suggests that even tightened muscles with no direct connection to the larynx can increase laryngeal tension. The commonest culprits are in the head and neck area: excess tension in the tongue, the jaw, or the neck. Singers who clench or grind their teeth or who have malocclusion, abnormal chewing habits, or symptomatic jaw dysfunction often have difficulty fully relaxing the laryngeal muscles. As already mentioned, tongue tie, and resultant tongue tension, is a recently recognized newcomer to the list of suspects.

Now let's look at some less obvious areas of tension that may cause vocal tension. Neck and shoulder tension are important and may have many causes. Apart from medical conditions such as arthritis or soft tissue injury after a car accident, many of us habitually carry tension in the mantle area.

Neck tightness due to a poor sitting or singing posture or just from stress is common. There is also an automatic tendency to pull in our necks and shrug our shoulders when stressed, frightened, or surprised. The startle response of pulling the shoulders up and the head down is reflexive, and its deconstruction and elimination is at the crux of the Alexander method for relaxing this area by consciously controlling and realigning the head, neck, and torso. Some people don't just startle but are in a chronic state of neck and shoulder tension. We can often tell whether a patient is left-handed or right-handed just by palpating the trapezius muscles. We spend more and more time huddled over our computers and cradling our phones against our ears, which can cause muscle strain. Heavy bags also pull on these muscles and cause a chronic contraction in the shoulder that bears the burden. Singers whose day jobs require carrying around laptops or documents (and yes, even those heavy scores and big bottles of water!) often have chronic tension in the neck and shoulder area.

Here are some simple suggestions. Declutter your bag frequently, taking only what you need for the day ahead. Use a bigger bag with a broad strap that you can sling diagonally across from the other shoulder. This distributes the weight more evenly to both sides and places the load closer to the center of your body, reducing torque. The most ergonomic arrangement is the "wineskin" bag that hugs the hollow of your waist on one side and is slung across your other shoulder. Another helpful option is a backpack with straps left long, so the load sits in the small of your back and rests on your sacral area. At the risk of looking like a bag lady, it may be better to carry two smaller bags in your two hands rather than one big one. And all else failing, consider one of those cheesy little wheeled bags/cases that paralegals and attorneys drag around. This takes the weight off your shoulders completely.

Sometimes even more distant and unconnected sources of muscle tension can have a negative impact. We have seen increased laryngeal tension in singers with lower back pain that may be due to nothing more than wearing high heels or standing on a steeply raked stage. Curvature of the upper back (thoracic scoliosis), a mild but relatively common condition more often seen in young women, can affect posture, breathing, and muscle tension. At times, patients have legs of uneven lengths, with a compensated posture that involves a pelvic tilt and increased resting muscle tone. Even transient abdominal and pelvic issues such as intestinal cramps, urinary tract infection, or painful periods can affect the voice, in addition to raising tension in the abdominal and pelvic floor muscles.

Case Report

A 25-year-old baritone presented with chronic hoarseness and persistent discomfort on the left side of his neck. Reflux was suspected, but initial treatment was only partially successful. Re-evaluation revealed left-sided neck tension, with tightness of the sternocleidomastoid muscle and elevation of the left shoulder (Fig 7.5). The cause was identified as a previously unsuspected curvature of the spine (scoliosis), and his symptoms improved with laryngeal massage and physical therapy.

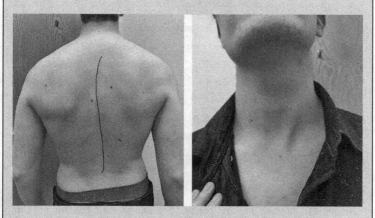

Figure 7.5 A previously undiagnosed thoracic scoliosis (left) caused asymmetric muscle tension in the left neck and muscle tension dysphonia in this singer.

Comment

When vocal muscle tension is identified, it is important to thoroughly search for its cause, which may be local or distant. Incorrectly attributing laryngeal muscle tension to the wrong cause not only will delay correct treatment but also may lead to further problems due to the wrong treatment.

The impact of distant muscle tension on the voice varies greatly from one person to another. Many singers have learned to overcome this and sing well despite ongoing musculoskeletal problems. Since stage performances in most vocal genres have become increasingly "athletic," being able to dissociate laryngeal function from muscle effort elsewhere in the body is important and the sign of a well-trained professional.

Case Report

A 40-year-old tenor presented with vocal difficulties while performing in Europe. He was seen by a local doctor who found a small swelling on one vocal fold. It was recommended that he cancel his performance and undergo surgery to remove the swelling. He did not follow this suggestion and completed his performances, although with some difficulty.

On his return, he related that he had fallen and injured his right arm and shoulder a few days before his first performance. He had considerable pain in the arm and had to sing with his arm immobilized against his chest. Examination further revealed severe muscle tension in the larynx and the neck. The neck muscles on the side of the arm injury were contracted and tender, and his larynx was visibly shifted to that side. Once the tension was addressed, his voice returned to normal. The small swelling also resolved, with no further treatment.

Comment

This case illustrates how the larynx, and the voice, can be impaired by muscle tension elsewhere in the body. In retrospect, the swelling was probably related to singing with abnormally heightened muscle tension.

In summary, tension in the vocal tract has many possible causes, ranging from the obvious (inadequate or inappropriate technical preparation) to more distant and seemingly unrelated, such as asymmetries in stance or posture. Recognizing the problem is an obvious first step. When searching for factors that increase laryngeal tension, a thorough review of musculoskeletal problems in other areas of the body is often helpful. It is also not uncommon to find more than one such focus, each one affecting general, and laryngeal, muscle tone to a different degree. You can check for laryngeal tension yourself by palpating the neck and with the glissando test. If the MTD follows specific episodes of vocal overuse, you should be able to correct it with vocal rest and appropriate vocal exercises. If, however, it persists, you should consider some of the other possible contributing factors, as outlined above.

8

Frequent Complaints, Common-Sense Solutions

One lesson we have learned from our singer patients is to take every complaint seriously. There is a tendency for all of us to dismiss things we don't understand as irrelevant or trivial. For doctors, this means that if a symptom does not fit with what we know or does not support the diagnosis we want to make, we tend to downplay it. This is understandable: we are all most comfortable with, and protective of, our knowledge base. We like every piece of the puzzle to fit.

With singers especially, it is difficult to fully share our patients' experience. What does it mean if a certain pitch "feels funny"? It is easier to deal with symptoms that have a clear physical correlate, something we can see or at least palpate. But all complaints need to be considered in context. Symptoms that may be temporary or trivial to nonsingers are potentially disastrous to a patient with an upcoming engagement or recording.

In this section, we address some of the most common medical complaints that singers experience. The list is not comprehensive, merely a brief overview, with a focus on how these problems affect singers and the singing voice. Please construe our advice as suggestions only: they are not meant to diagnose your specific problems. As always, when in doubt, you need to consult your own doctor.

Keep Your Singing Voice Healthy! Anthony F. Jahn and Youngnan Jenny Cho, Oxford University Press.
© Oxford University Press 2024. DOI: 10.1093/9780197629703.003.0008

Mucus: Too Much or Too Little?

High on the list of "trivial but serious" problems is mucus. Mucus in the back of the nose or throat, on the vocal folds, or in the chest can be a chronic and frustrating problem. What is mucus, and how do we deal with it?

Most of the vocal tract, from the smallest connections in the lungs to the nose, is covered by mucous membrane. Since these interior passages are not exposed to the wear and tear of the outside world, they have evolved a self-cleaning mechanism to remove any debris or unnecessary material. And mucus plays a key role.

Mucus is a clear viscous fluid secreted by tiny flask-shaped cells embedded in the mucous membrane. Once secreted, mucus normally spreads over the surface in a thin layer that coats the respiratory (and vocal) tract. Unlike water (or watery saliva), the molecules of mucus are large and complex. Most importantly, they are cross-linked, forming a three-dimensional mesh "blanket" that covers the lining of the vocal tract. A second population of cells in the membrane, equipped with tiny hairlike projections (cilia), is tasked with moving the mucous blanket along. The tips of the cilia protrude up into the lower layer of the mucous sheet and, ratchetlike, propel it along the surface.

Day and night, a thin film of mucus is constantly streaming in a slow-motion cascade, from the inside of the sinuses, the bronchi, and the trachea. Like a conveyor belt, the mucus carries along inhaled dust particles, pollen, and even bacteria. The speed and efficiency of this mucus-moving machine (the "mucociliary escalator") varies greatly and depends on many factors, some of which are discussed below. The process slows down at night when we sleep, which may account for an apparent excess of mucus in the morning, requiring throat clearing in a hot shower. However, it remains in constant motion throughout our lives—it even continues for a few hours after death!

Like all roads leading to Rome, all the streams of mucus have a common destination: the back of the throat. The cilia in the bronchi and trachea beat upward, the cilia in the sinuses beat toward the inside of the nose, and the cilia in the nose beat backward, but all mucus eventually ends in the hypopharynx at the entrance to the esophagus, presenting the perennial dilemma: spit or swallow?

Our bodies normally produce about one to two quarts of mucus a day, much of which we swallow unawares. If mucus is the right amount and the right consistency, its presence goes unnoticed. We become aware only when the mucus is too much or too thick, or its flow is impeded.

In addition to trapping debris and clearing the airway, mucus keeps the membranes moist. It also has a protective function and tends to adhere to areas of inflammation. Interestingly, the vocal folds are the only part of the vocal tract *not* covered by a mucus-producing membrane. The folds are moistened indirectly: mucous glands in the laryngeal ventricles above trickle thin mucus down onto the surface of the vocal folds.

Excess Mucus

With respiratory tract infections such as a cold, rhinitis, sinusitis, tracheitis, or bronchitis, the body produces more mucus in protective response. The mucus is also thicker, often containing bacteria or pus. This higher-viscosity material can overwhelm normal ciliary transport, requiring us to clear our throats or cough.

Allergies are another group of conditions to be considered. Inhalant allergies cause nasal irritation and sneezing, but food allergies may only cause a low-grade inflammation of the pharynx with excessively adherent mucus. Dairy products can cause excess mucus even in the absence of a specific allergy.

FREQUENT COMPLAINTS, COMMON-SENSE SOLUTIONS 77

In fact, local inflammation from any cause makes mucus more adherent. Even excessive singing, causing minimal temporary irritation of the vocal folds, may cause bits of mucus to stick to their surface. Irritated vocal nodules are often covered by a small drop of mucus, which needs to be cleared before the larynx can be fully examined.

If a patient complains of feeling mucus in the absence of any obvious inflammation, there is often not too much mucus, but too little. The mucus may be scant but dry, and hence it cannot be easily cleared. When it becomes too thick, the cilia get gummed up and can no longer propel it along the surface.

As mentioned above, mucus adheres to inflamed membranes. Patients with pharyngeal irritation from acid reflux commonly feel mucus in the throat, and constant throat clearing is one feature of silent reflux. The inflammation need not be severe for mucus to stick to these surfaces. Mucus may also accumulate in the nose or sinus passages if these areas are inflamed.

An infrequent but frequently overlooked cause of adherent mucus in the hypopharynx is yeast infection. We see this mostly in asthmatic patients who use a steroid inhaler, but also in others who have taken prednisone or prolonged or repeated courses of antibiotics. Food allergies may also cause thick mucus, most likely due to inflamed mucous membranes that have been in contact with triggering foods.

And finally, consider the possibility that excess mucus accumulation may be due not only to overproduction but also impaired clearing. Respiratory cilia become less effective with age, as well as due to environmental toxins. Nicotine slows mucus clearance by paralyzing the cilia. When this is the problem, mucus will accumulate not just in the nose and throat but also in the trachea and bronchi. On the other hand, if a patient has difficulty with mucus accumulation just in the nose, narrowed nasal passages should also be considered. Common causes for this include obstruction from a deviated nasal septum or swollen turbinates.

Inadequate Mucus

Excessive dryness can also impair normal function of the vocal tract. When the mucous membranes are dry, they are unable to trap and clear inhaled particles such as pollen or other allergens. These irritants then travel deeper into the respiratory tract and can cause more severe allergic symptoms. In such cases the mucus produced is often more viscous and unable to efficiently lubricate and protect the lining of the vocal tract. For the singer, excessive dryness of the vocal folds makes them less pliable and impairs phonation, especially when singing softly at the top of the range.

The causes for inadequate mucus and vocal "dryness" are numerous. They include inadequate water intake, inadequate ambient humidity, and smoking and other irritant exposure. With age there is also a general decrease in normal mucus formation, so dryness may occur. When mucus dries, it tends to clump and accumulate, leading to postnasal drip and throat clearing. Many medications (such as antidepressants) can be drying. Inappropriate use of antihistamines may also dry the throat and impair the voice. This is an important point, since patients who experience "excess mucus" (in reality, mucus that is inadequate but viscous) will often try to treat themselves with antihistamines, causing further dryness and worsening their symptoms. Take note of when the problem occurs: Is it during high allergy season? Is it in conjunction with certain medications? Or is it part of performance anxiety? The ideal management involves identifying the cause first.

Mucus Relief

There are several measures that can help with troublesome mucus. First, adequate hydration! Most doctors recommend drinking eight 8-oz. glasses of water a day, but how can you keep count? The easiest method is to drink two glasses with each meal, and one

FREQUENT COMPLAINTS, COMMON-SENSE SOLUTIONS 79

glass between meals $(2 + 1 + 2 + 1 + 2 = 8)$. Water or herbal tea is the best. Remember to further increase your hydration if you are dehydrating yourself with vigorous exercise, alcohol consumption, or medications or during hot weather.

If the mucus originates from the nose (postnasal drip), consider the possibility of increased mucus production (nasal allergies or sinusitis) or impaired mucus transport. Wash your nose once or twice a day with warm salt water. There are several devices available for this, the simplest being a neti pot. More aggressive washing, using a squeeze bottle or a suction-irrigation device, are also effective. If the nasal passages are not obstructed, this should adequately clean the mucous membranes. If the nasal mucus is particularly thick, try adding a drop of baby shampoo to the neti pot once in a while (stir with your finger—don't shake it). The drop of soap works at the molecular level to break up substances that are not normally water soluble. If mucus still continues to accumulate in the back of the nose, consider the possibility of a blocked or narrowed nasal passage, especially if you are also aware of obstructed nasal breathing, snoring, or recurrent sinus infections.

Inhaling steam through the nose and mouth also helps to moisturize (and mobilize) the mucus. Remember, the cilia cannot move the mucous blanket if they are gummed up by dry secretions or overwhelmed by excessive quantities of mucus on the surface.

Increasing ambient air moisture is particularly important in a dry environment (such as a desert climate) and in the winter if your home is heated. We recommend a humidifier, at least for your bedroom, and ideally for the entire dwelling. A cool-air humidifier works best—hot steam rises to the ceiling. Nebulizers generate much smaller particles of moisture and are not necessary unless you have bronchial or pulmonary problems or you need to inhale a medication. Nasal dryness can be treated with an over-the-counter (OTC) saline gel spray, which coats the membranes and prevents drying longer than a simple saline water spray. These last two suggestions are often also helpful in controlling inhalant allergies such as dust.

If mucus develops in conjunction with certain foods, such as dairy, try a four-week elimination diet. Remove the food, or class of foods, that may be responsible from your meals. Not to sound contrarian, but milk is not especially "good for you"! Milk is a bovine glandular secretion meant for calves that has been oversold by the dairy industry. Try substituting soy or almond milk and reducing high-fat milk products (like cheeses), and consider adding other calcium-rich foods, such as legumes, nuts, and seeds, to your diet. If you see a correlation between food and mucus but cannot identify the culprit, consult a doctor who offers food allergy testing.

Oral medications, such as **guaifenesin** or **n-acetyl cysteine**, can greatly help to loosen mucus, but these only work in the presence of adequate hydration. If you travel internationally, n-acetyl cysteine is available in many European pharmacies as an effervescent tablet you dissolve in water and then drink. In the US, it is an OTC pill or capsule, but you may need to order it online. It breaks up mucus by disrupting the cross-linking molecular bonds that make mucus viscous. However you manage your mucus problems, remember, whether too much or too little, the foundation of mucus management is generous and constant hydration.

Throat Infections

These are usually caused by bacteria or viruses. Their onset may be accompanied by some coldlike symptoms, even a slight fever. The back of the throat (oropharynx) is diffusely sore, and the inflammation is usually localized to the pharynx.

Most throat infections don't extend to the vocal folds. On the other hand, irritation of the hypopharynx can increase muscle tension during phonation. With severe infections such as bacterial tonsillitis, the voice may sound covered or muffled. If the tonsils

FREQUENT COMPLAINTS, COMMON-SENSE SOLUTIONS 81

are very swollen, they can partly occlude the oropharynx, causing a "hot potato" voice.

If you look in the back of your sore throat with a flashlight, you might see diffuse redness and swelling of the membranes. The tonsils can also be swollen, at times covered with white spots. Both bacterial and viral infections can make it difficult to swallow, especially solids.

It can be difficult to distinguish bacterial from viral sore throats. Here are some clues: Bacterial infections tend to be more severe and may be accompanied by tender swollen lymph nodes in the upper neck. If the tonsils have small white spots on them, the infection is usually bacterial. Viral infections may cause small blisters on the palate or in the throat. One condition that goes against these rules is infectious mononucleosis: although viral, it causes multiple nodes in the neck, and the tonsils can appear white, covered by an infected membrane.

Rapid culture of the throat is not always accurate, especially when trying to rule out strep infections. These cultures may miss the strep and do not identify several other types of bacteria that also need treatment. We have both seen singers with bacterial pharyngitis who were (incorrectly) told that they do not need antibiotics because the instant strep test was negative.

Home remedies? Gargling with warm saltwater is useful. The solution should be hypertonic, slightly higher in salt than the normal isotonic solution used for nasal washing. The increased salt decreases the swelling by drawing fluid out of the swollen tissues. Warm tea with honey also helps: the heat increases blood flow to the area, hastening healing, and the honey (like the salt) creates a hypertonic solution that reduces localized swelling and pain. Exposing bacteria to a hypertonic solution, whether salt or sugar, can reduce their number. Our personal favorite is warm ginger tea with manuka honey, made with fresh ginger boiled in water. While a bit spicy, this can significantly reduce throat pain. Some studies suggest that ginger additionally acts as a mucus thinner and a bronchodilator, so it's good all around! Finally, the use of OTC pain medications such as acetaminophen or ibuprofen will also help. If the pain continues and your symptoms worsen, however, you will need to see a doctor and may need antibiotics.

Tonsillitis

The tonsils are two almond-shaped structures that sit on either side of the oropharynx, at the junction of the tongue and the soft palate. Like the two armed men in Mozart's "Magic Flute," they guard the entrance to the throat and, in early childhood, play an important role in generating antibodies against infections. Their job is mostly completed by age four, however, and as a child grows older, tonsils lose most of their function and normally atrophy. They have a minimal immune-protective role in adulthood.

In young adults, persistent tonsils may cause problems in two ways. If they remain large, they can partly obstruct the airway and cause snoring. At night our muscles relax, and tonsils flip-flop back and forth more easily as we breathe, especially if we sleep in a supine position. For singers, enlarged tonsils can partly occlude the oropharynx, creating a covered voice. If massively enlarged, tonsils can also weigh down the soft palate, making it more difficult to lift during singing.

A second problem is recurrent infection. In this scenario, the tonsils may not be very large, but they have become chronically infected. Colonies of bacteria live within the tonsil tissue all the time. Standard doses of antibiotics may not fully kill such bacteria since the colonies are surrounded by scar tissue that limits tissue penetration of medications. The bugs are normally kept quiet by the immune system; however, when the immunity is temporarily impaired, the bacteria become symptomatic. Clinically, this manifests as recurrent sore throats, which respond to, but are never fully cured by, antibiotics.

FREQUENT COMPLAINTS, COMMON-SENSE SOLUTIONS   83

That temporary decrease in immunity may be caused by many factors, including a concurrent infection elsewhere, overexertion, and even emotional stress. Not coincidentally, these young adults often get tonsillitis before a stressful examination or audition or during a personal crisis.

Tonsil stones are another manifestation of low-grade chronic infection. These little bits of bad-smelling cheesy debris form in the pockets (crypts) of the tonsil, causing bad breath. They can usually be dislodged with a long cotton swab (or a long probing fingernail) but will recur intermittently, as your immunity level fluctuates.

Although antibiotics, a strong immune system, and stress management are helpful, it is our recommendation that if tonsils cause chronic problems, they should be removed. Surgery can be done with minimal trauma, taking care to maximally preserve normal tissues, by someone who is familiar with the anatomic requirements of singers. Done correctly, the voice will not be affected and, equally important, the patient's general health status will improve.

Nasal Obstruction

The nose (not the mouth) is the normal organ of respiration. It is designed to filter, heat, and humidify inhaled air. Nasal breathing also increases lung compliance, so we all should, if possible, breathe through our nose. The inside of the nose is divided into two cavities by the septum, a thin midline partition of cartilage and bone that runs vertically from the top of the nose to the floor, forming the medial wall of each nasal passage. The floor of the nose is the hard palate, and it transmits sound vibration into the nasal cavities as you sing. The outer wall of each nasal cavity is lined by three shelves of bone and soft tissue, the turbinates. These are the main heaters and humidifiers of inhaled air, and the large inferior turbinate is most important in this regard. The turbinates alternately swell and shrink in tandem fashion (called the vasomotor cycle of the nose), resulting in nasal airflow that alternates from one side to the other. At any time, we typically breathe more easily through one side of the nose.

Intermittent mild nasal blockage is normal; however, persistent nasal obstruction can become a problem, particularly for singers. Apart from not being able to breathe normally, singers with nasal blockage may have an altered sensation of bone-conducted sound when they sing. The open nose is a significant resonator for the voice, and patients with a constantly blocked nose may have difficulty achieving nasal and facial proprioception in the head register. When nasal obstruction is corrected, our patients tell us that the voice comes forward and flips more easily into the mask.

Chronic nasal obstruction prevents normal nasal airflow. Common causes are a deviation of the septum and overgrowth of the inferior turbinates. If the septum is not straight but curved or buckled, it protrudes into the nasal cavity, blocking airflow. When the turbinates are enlarged, they obstruct the nasal passage. Less commonly, chronic infection or nasal polyps may block the nose.

How can you tell, short of a doctor's visit, whether you have nasal obstruction? Occlude one nostril and breathe in, and then repeat on the other side. Do you feel, or hear, more resistance? Repeat several times over the day. If the blockage remains on the same side, you may have a problem. You can also try the speech therapist's trick of exhaling through your nose onto a polished hand mirror and noting which side fogs up the mirror less.

Snoring is a common sign of nasal obstruction (although there are other causes as well). Why do we snore? When the nose is open, inhaled air flows smoothly in a laminar fashion. With areas of obstruction, the flow becomes turbulent, forming eddies of air current. The turbulence generates vibrations in the palate and pharynx, which become audible. If the nasal air intake is insufficient, patients need to breathe through the mouth, adding to the cacophony.

FREQUENT COMPLAINTS, COMMON-SENSE SOLUTIONS   85

If you have difficulties moving the voice into the mask, consider that you may have a degree of nasal obstruction. Is it inflammation or a structural problem? Try a decongestant nasal spray to see if the obstruction resolves: simple swelling, such as from allergies or a cold, should respond, while a fixed obstruction, as from a deviated septum, will not. If some blockage persists, a visit to your doctor may be in order to correct the deviation and restore full nasal resonance to your voice.

Sinusitis

The sinuses are air-filled cavities that surround the nose. The major sinuses are in both cheeks (maxillary), over the forehead (frontal), and between the eyes (ethmoid). A deeper set is behind the nose, at the base of the skull (sphenoid).

Sinuses develop as outpouchings from the nose and normally maintain their connection to the nose through small connecting passages. They are also lined with mucous membrane that is continuous with the mucous membrane in the nose. The function of sinuses is not clear. Some have suggested that they lighten the skull by hollowing it out or that they strengthen the facial skeleton. More recently, it has been shown that they produce a gas (nitrous oxide), which, when inhaled, may have a positive effect on lung function, another good reason to breathe nasally.

For singers, the sinuses are resonating chambers that provide a sensation of sound vibration "in the mask." This sensation indicates correct placement of the voice and is responsible for the term "head voice." Although this resonance is physically felt by the singer, it does not significantly enhance the sung voice as heard by others.

The mucous membrane linings of the nose and the sinuses form one contiguous surface. Since everything is connected, it makes sense that infections in the nose may spread to the sinuses. The problem arises when the small connecting openings become blocked. When the openings swell shut, they block the ventilation of the sinuses. Whether the blockage is due to infection, allergies, or other irritants, once the sinuses become blocked, symptoms may develop. The air pressure in the sinuses, normally the same as in the nose (and the outside), decreases, and pain develops. In the old days, this phenomenon was called "vacuum headaches," which is not a bad description for what happens. Since the self-cleansing mechanism is also interrupted, if there is a coexistent infection, soiled secretions become trapped in the sinuses.

Patients often describe a blocked and drippy nose as "sinuses," but sinusitis is quite different from rhinitis (nasal inflammation). Depending on which sinus is involved, infection causes pain and pressure, which can be felt over the cheeks (maxillary), between the eyes (ethmoid), and over the forehead (frontal). These areas may become tender when gently tapped. Since the sphenoid sinuses are not close to the surface, sphenoid sinusitis causes pain either at the top or at the back of the head. The roots of the posterior teeth protrude into the maxillary sinus, so toothache or pressure over the palate is another possible symptom. In most cases, as the nasal symptoms resolve, the sinuses also open and begin to drain. If the sinus pain persists or worsens, and especially if accompanied by fever, medical attention is required.

Management of early sinus symptoms, however, can be done at home, and here are some suggestions. Since the proximate cause is the blockage of sinus openings, you should try to decongest these areas. Topical decongestant sprays, such as Neo-Synephrine or oxymetazoline, are useful. These shrink the swollen turbinates and can re-establish sinus ventilation. You can also irrigate your nose with a neti pot, adding a few decongestant drops to the saline. This method more thoroughly reaches deeper nasal surfaces than a simple spray and can be more effective for sinus blockage.

Inhaling steam with one to two drops of eucalyptus oil added can also be beneficial, although the effect is not quite as dramatic as a medicated nasal spray. In general, we do not recommend steroid

FREQUENT COMPLAINTS, COMMON-SENSE SOLUTIONS 87

sprays (such as fluticasone) for nasal or sinus infections, since these are often not effective and may prolong an infection. Applying topical heat, using a moist warm towel, to your face will increase local circulation and can be done in addition to decongestant nasal sprays or washes.

Oral decongestants are also helpful. The most frequently used is pseudoephedrine (Sudafed). This acts like adrenaline and opens the nasal passages, decongesting the nasal lining and helping to relieve sinus pressure. Sudafed is often a part of many "cold and sinus" compounds. It has some side effects (dryness and increasing the heart rate) but is often useful for sinus pressure.

Of the various herbal remedies, our personal favorite is "Gouttes aux Essences," a preparation of drops combining extracts of clove, lavender, menthol, thyme, and cinnamon. It is manufactured by Naturactive Laboratoires (France) and available online. A few drops of this extract, taken orally in a glass of hot water, will often decongest the nose and sinuses without the side effects of conventional medications. Of course, analgesics (Tylenol or Advil) are useful adjuncts but do not directly open the sinuses.

Most cases of mild acute sinusitis resolve spontaneously. The treatment suggestions above are simply for the management of sinus pain and obstruction; they do not treat the underlying cause, whether infection or allergy. If you get recurrent sinus infections or if every cold progresses to sinusitis, you should consider a medical evaluation and possibly a computed tomography scan to see whether there is a predisposing anatomic abnormality.

If you need to perform while experiencing sinusitis, here are a couple of suggestions. Use a nasal decongestant spray before singing to reduce any nasal blockage and help to open the sinuses. If there is a lot of mucus in addition to congestion, wash your nose using a squeeze bottle filled with saline that has six drops of decongestant added. This will both clean your nose and open the passages. If the sinusitis is not due to infection or if the infection is also being treated with antibiotics, a short course of prednisone will decrease your sinus symptoms. Keep in mind, however, that prednisone interferes with your body's ability to rid itself of an infection. This option should only be used in an emergency and in conjunction with antibiotics. We also suggest that you avoid the all-in-one cold and sinus compounds, since they contain other medications (antihistamines, pain and cough suppressants) that you may not need, and that can cause dryness sensation.

Throat Discomfort after Singing

A throat ache from vocal strain is the singer's equivalent to the athlete's pulled muscles. It can occur after extensive singing, singing under suboptimal conditions (as with an overamplified backup band or at times of impaired health), or singing material that is beyond the performer's capabilities, either because it is unsuitable or because the singer lacks adequate training. Performing under these circumstances can cause muscle tension dysphonia, which we discussed earlier. However, it can also cause throat ache.

The distinguishing features of such discomfort are clear. It occurs after prolonged vocal strain, usually the following morning. Unlike infections, the pain is not severe, more of an ache. It is localized to the area of the larynx, not the back of the throat. You can often point to the area of discomfort in the neck, and the area may be tender to pressure. The adjacent neck muscles may also be tender and cramped, especially the muscles above the larynx. The voice may be slightly hoarse, but not muffled, as with throat infections. The glissando test may reveal hoarseness in head voice, as well as a defect in the register shift. Unlike with infections, throat pain from laryngeal strain does not impair swallowing.

Managing Vocal Strain

Prolonged performance singing (versus singing to yourself in the shower) is effortful and strenuous, even if done with perfect technique. A vocal performance of any significance should normally be followed by a period of relative vocal rest. This is a time when the larynx is recovering, the vocal folds are moving gently to and fro with each breath, and the muscles are in a state of relaxation, contracting only intermittently with the occasional swallow. Even when there is no discomfort after a performance, resting the vocal apparatus makes sense. Vocal rest is covered in greater detail elsewhere in this book.

However, if you consistently get throat discomfort after singing, you need to analyze why. Some healthy muscle fatigue after prolonged singing is acceptable, but recurrent pain and tenderness suggest that you need to change your behavior. While your teacher is your best guide in this regard, here are some suggestions.

First, avoid (if you can) excessively long practice sessions. Shorter, more frequent, and problem-focused practicing is kinder to your throat. Mindful practicing is addressed in a subsequent chapter.

If you need to sing while not at your best (premenstrual, dealing with a cold, allergies, or other problems), cut yourself some slack rather than trying to "power through." If practicing, work instead on other aspects, such as memorizing. If performing, consider your environment, the venue, the other performers (instrumental or choral), the amplification system, and other factors.

The simple remedy for pain from vocal strain is vocal rest. Do not sing, and reduce speaking to a soft and essential minimum. Remember that while the strain may have come from singing, even speaking can interfere with recovery. Avoid exercise to reduce further muscle strain: you will recall that contracting muscles anywhere in the body can heighten the resting tone in every muscle, including the larynx. Breathing through the nose humidifies the inhaled air, increases the flexibility of the lungs, and allows the vocal folds to gently open and close with each breath, providing a light massaging effect.

90   KEEP YOUR SINGING VOICE HEALTHY!

While recovering from vocal strain, we also recommend that you avoid listening to loud music. Loud music (or sound) causes our ears to prepare the larynx to speak loudly. Even without phonating, the muscles tighten, which is the opposite of what vocal rest aims to achieve.

Laryngeal massage is a good adjunct to vocal rest. If you are unable to do this yourself and do not have access to someone who does, treat yourself to a good massage of the back and neck. These areas adjacent to the vocal tract are often also tight, and by relaxing them, vocal strain and the associated discomfort will dissipate faster. Acupuncture can also help to relax tense muscles.

There are two more points relating to pain associated with oversinging. If, along with pain and tenderness, your voice has become hoarse and the hoarseness persists beyond the time when your other symptoms have resolved, you should have your larynx examined. Vocal fold hemorrhage, while in itself painless, may occur in the context of excessive strain. If this happens, it needs to be identified and managed.

Finally, at the risk of repetition, if throat discomfort after singing is a common phenomenon for you, you need to take a serious look at what you are doing wrong. Unlike throat pain from infections, discomfort after singing is a self-inflicted problem that you need to solve before causing structural damage to the vocal folds.

Acid Reflux

Acid reflux seems to be an increasingly frequent condition. Has it become the affliction of our times? Some would say so—we eat hurriedly, at odd times, and often too much. We often don't know what we're eating, picking up food made by "persons unknown" in the back room of a restaurant or store, and containing ingredients we cannot identify. On the run and under stress, we do not pay

FREQUENT COMPLAINTS, COMMON-SENSE SOLUTIONS 91

enough attention to what, when, and how we eat. The result is acid reflux.

Is it just reflux, or reflux disease? Reflux means that stomach contents, acid and enzymes, travel back up the esophagus. This occasionally happens to all of us with no consequence. However, when the acid refluxes frequently or excessively, it can cause problems. The irritating fluid can reach the lower parts of the pharynx but may on occasion travel even higher. It is then that simple occasional reflux acquires the more ominous title of gastroesophageal reflux *disease* (GERD). Reflux is the cause; GERD is the result.

GERD can cause several troublesome symptoms for the singer. One frequent complaint is **throat pain**, usually felt in the hypopharynx. Typically, there is a sore throat in the morning, which resolves later in the day. This occurs if you have reflux at night, when you are lying flat, making that trip up the esophagus easier, horizontal, and not vertical.

This morning throat pain is different from a dry throat that might develop if you, say, sleep with the mouth open. It is lower in the throat and often localized to one side. If the side of the pain is the same as the side you sleep on, nocturnal reflux is the likely cause. If you aren't sure which side you sleep on, consider this question: which side do you wake up on? If pain and sleeping position are both on the same side, you may have made a diagnosis of nocturnal reflux. Throat pain from reflux may also cause an earache on the same side. Although earache can occur with infections also, if it is unilateral (on the same side), that is a significant clue.

While definitive diagnosis and treatment may require a medical visit, if you suspect GERD, you can try a simple experiment: elevate the top end of your bed and take a liquid antacid before going to bed at night. You can elevate the head of your bed by placing a couple of thick books or bricks under the feet or by placing a wedge under the top end of the mattress. Do not raise your head by using extra pillows, as you might get neck strain. If the throat pain resolves, the diagnosis is pretty clear. If, however, the pain recurs or persists, you will need an examination, since there are other potentially serious conditions that may present with unilateral throat pain.

A sensation of **excessive mucus and throat clearing** may also be due to GERD. Remember that when mucous membranes are inflamed, they generate more mucus, and the mucus becomes more adherent. Not surprisingly, when the hypopharynx is bathed in gastric juices, it becomes irritated. The excess mucus can interfere with singing and triggers the need to frequently clear the throat. If you have these symptoms, you should suspect reflux, especially if mucus and throat clearing are associated with certain foods or if your eating habits (times, duration, quantity, and nature of your food) are such that reflux may result.

A simple initial approach would be to change how you approach your meals. Eliminate potential food culprits, such as dairy or high-reflux foods such as tomatoes. Try to eat smaller meals more frequently, like our foraging ancestors. Eat your evening meal earlier and make it smaller. Reduce coffee and alcohol. More ambitiously, lose excess weight: even a few pounds can reduce the abdominal pressure that pushes gastric contents upward. Consider this as an experiment and give yourself a couple of months: if excessive mucus and throat clearing decrease, you're on the right track. If they are still a problem, then you should see a doctor for evaluation and treatment.

Yet another feature of reflux is a **change of voice.** Singers with GERD commonly lose vocal flexibility and clarity. Depending on the amount and frequency of reflux, the voice may become significantly impaired. An obvious connection in this regard is if your voice is hoarse after reflux-triggering events. Morning hoarseness that does not easily clear with a hot and steamy shower is suggestive. If you drink excessive amounts of coffee, reflux may become more frequent, since coffee relaxes the sphincter separating the esophagus and the stomach.

FREQUENT COMPLAINTS, COMMON-SENSE SOLUTIONS 93

A lot has been written on how reflux "damages the voice," much of which is misleading. The truth is that most of the vocal change is not due to actual laryngeal damage and is easily reversed with correct treatment. The effect of GERD on the voice is mostly indirect: inflammation of the pharynx causes irritation and contraction of the surrounding muscles and elevation of the larynx. Much like muscle tension dysphonia, the larynx in GERD patients is in the wrong position, its muscles contracting with excess tension. In fact, the commonest voice problem we see in GERD patients is in the middle voice, around the register shift.

And this is confirmed on examination: while there is often inflammation of tissues around the vocal folds (and between the folds posteriorly), the vocal folds themselves usually appear normal and are very rarely irritated. We emphasize this point to counter such overdramatizing comments as "your vocal folds are burned," which are not only unnecessarily frightening but also factually incorrect. In fact, **while reflux-induced laryngeal tension is quite common, actual damage to the vocal folds is rare.** This means that with proper GERD treatment, the voice usually recovers with no lasting effects to the vocal folds or the voice.

The management of reflux can take many forms. Obviously losing weight, if appropriate, should be considered, as well as avoiding dietary triggers and eating schedules. A variety of medications are also available, both by prescription and OTC, which reduce acid secretion, neutralize stomach acid, and block the regurgitation of acid up the esophagus. If your reflux symptoms persist despite a trial of OTC remedies, it is best to consult a physician for further management. As a side note, remember that some Alka Seltzer preparations contain aspirin, which may not be necessary for you and can have additional potential side effects.

A couple of final thoughts: due to the prevalence of reflux, the attribution of hoarseness to GERD has become the diagnostic darling of many physicians, often incorrectly so. We frequently see refluxing singers who sing perfectly well, others with no reflux

94   KEEP YOUR SINGING VOICE HEALTHY!

who are hoarse, and still others who remain hoarse even after their GERD is eliminated. Giving such patients more and more antireflux medications is barking up the wrong tree. If vocal difficulties persist after an appropriate trial of antireflux treatment, you may need to consider other possible causes.

But if persistent throat pain, cough, or difficulty swallowing persists, you need to see a physician for further evaluation.

Headache

Books have been written on this topic, but we briefly would like to give some direction for those who experience head pain. Certainly, if the headache is recurrent, progressive, or severe, you need to see a doctor. Severe, sudden-onset headache for no apparent cause requires immediate medical attention.

Here are some common-sense initial directions, however. The simplest distinction is to consider where the pain occurs. Pain or pressure over the face (forehead, between the eyes, or cheeks) is most likely related to the sinuses. If you have sinusitis, gently tapping over the area might feel tender. Sinus pain is often associated with nasal blockage or excessive nasal discharge. If the discharge is colored (yellow or green), you should suspect a bacterial infection. If cheek pain is on one side only, you should consider a dental problem, a frequent cause of unilateral sinusitis. Home remedies for sinusitis include oral and topical decongestants and saline irrigation of the nose, described earlier in this chapter.

The quality of the pain is also a significant clue. Pressure or throbbing is usually due to inflammation, such as sinusitis. Sharp shooting pain may be nerve related, such as dental pain. A chronic low-grade discomfort may be a sign of muscle cramping. While these are clues, they are not in themselves diagnostic.

Headache on top or in the back of the head may be related to elevated blood pressure. If you are hypertensive or suspect you may

FREQUENT COMPLAINTS, COMMON-SENSE SOLUTIONS   95

be, invest in a blood pressure cuff and monitor your blood pressure regularly. Pain over the temples or in the upper neck is frequently due to tension. Tension in the neck muscles often causes pain where these muscles insert into the back of the skull. Finger pressure over these cramped muscles can elicit tenderness. Muscle tension over the temples is often due to jaw clenching or grinding the teeth: the temporal muscles, the main muscles that close (and clench) the jaw, attach here, above the ears. Habitual or excessive clenching can also cause pain in front of the ears, where the jaw joint (temporo-mandibular joint [TMJ]) is. By firmly pressing in this area while you open and close your mouth, you can see whether there is tenderness over this area. Grinding or clicking that you can feel with the fingers pressed over the TMJ is another clue that the jaw is not working properly.

There are of course many other causes of head and facial pain, including migraines and neuralgia, some potentially serious, and you may need to see your doctor to sort these out and find effective treatment, especially if the pain is sudden in onset, is severe, persists, or progresses.

Hoarseness

This is perhaps the most significant complaint among our singer patients: in a sense, this whole book is about hoarseness, loss of the ability to phonate normally and easily. While we cannot cover every cause of hoarseness, a few practical points should be considered.

First, hoarseness is a terribly nonspecific term. For nonsingers it may suffice, just meaning that the voice is raspy, not normal. But singers hear, feel, measure, and generally hold their voice to a higher standard, and for this group, a "voice that is not normal" comes in dozens of varieties. Since most singers vocalize every day, they perform a daily painstaking and focused diagnostic checkup that looks at every aspect of their instrument. The abnormalities they hear may affect the singing voice but not the speaking voice. The problem may affect the entire vocal range, occurring only in specific registers or at the transition points. There may be a loss of notes on the top, breathiness, muffling or a loss of resonance. The change may be insignificant to the outside listener but obvious to the critical ear of the singer.

How to approach a voice that is not normal? Before you rush to a doctor, there is actually quite a lot you can do to get a sense of what may be wrong. We have already covered self-examination of the larynx and the **glissando test**, which allows your critical ear to dissect the voice and identify specific problems through your vocal range. But to get a better picture, you need to ask yourself some questions that will more accurately diagnose your problem.

First, what is the time and mode of onset? Did you experience hoarseness first thing in the morning, or after prolonged singing? Did it just happen suddenly, for no reason, or develop gradually over weeks or months? Can you link it to outdoor activity during allergy season, excessive voice use, or your menstrual cycle? Hoarseness in the morning may be just "morning voice," a combination of dryness and mucus accumulation that will clear after a long steamy shower and gentle vocalization. It might also be due to nocturnal mouth breathing if your nose is obstructed. Finally, consider gastric reflux, which can occur if you are overweight, eat late at night, or drink alcohol with dinner. Hoarseness after prolonged singing may be due to mild swelling of the vocal folds. This is more likely if the singing was effortful, if you're underhydrated and the folds are dry, or if you are singing over a cold, infection, or other physical impairment.

Sudden change in the voice that occurs with physical effort, vocal or otherwise, could be the sign of vocal hemorrhage, discussed in more detail elsewhere. In addition to effortful singing, we have seen vocal hemorrhage occur with weightlifting, straining (bearing down), paroxysms of cough, loud yelling, and prolonged vomiting. In women, this is more likely to happen during menstruation,

FREQUENT COMPLAINTS, COMMON-SENSE SOLUTIONS   97

and it is overall more common in those who take blood thinners. In this regard, consider that some supplements, such as gingko and Chinese tree ear mushroom, can thin the blood or open the circulation.

Did your voice suddenly become hoarse, for no apparent reason? This is a tricky one. Certainly a virus can cause vocal fold weakness, with no other symptoms, although you may experience some coexisting signs of a viral infection. But consider that some cases of hoarseness appear to be sudden in onset when they are not. This is because trained singers can overcome mild impairment by adjusting their phonation unawares. With subtle technical modifications, such as muscling the voice a bit or singing with more support, the mild impairment may not manifest until vocal compensation is no longer adequate. At this point, compensation fails and the hoarseness appears, seemingly "suddenly."

If hoarseness is chronic and has not resolved with voice rest, is it fluctuating in severity, or is it always the same? Is it improving or worsening over time? This is a situation where you need to monitor the vocal status carefully, with daily glissando testing. Are notes progressively disappearing from the top? Is there more and more noise or air in the voice? Is the hoarseness progressing from head into chest range? Is it affecting both singing and speaking voice?

If your hoarseness is persistent, fluctuating in severity, recurrent, or progressive, you will need to be examined by your laryngologist. Many conditions can present in this fashion, including polyps, nodules, cysts, dilated blood vessels, or a variety of conditions, covered in more detail elsewhere in the book. If voice change is associated with other symptoms such as pain, impaired breathing, or swallowing, you need to be seen sooner rather than later.

9

A Practical Approach to Allergies

Allergies seem to be everywhere, and on the rise. Increasing ease and frequency of travel, the growing prevalence of worldwide importation of animals, foods, and other commodities, as well as climate change are just some of the causes. To illustrate the trend, consider just one example: only a few decades ago, allergy sufferers were exhorted to "Take your sinuses to Arizona!," then a dry, warm region with a few cacti for vegetation, a couple of lizards scurrying around the sand, and no allergies. Since then, a massive influx of northerners, bringing their flowering plants, hair-shedding pets, and other allergens, have put that slogan to rest.

Singers are particularly prone to allergies. Their schedule often involves traveling to different parts of the world with exposure to local flora and other allergens. Crossing time zones (and seasons) and spending time in a variety of environments increase the potential for allergic triggers. Stages (and especially backstages) are often dusty. They frequently serve as temporary storage areas for unused sets and props. Moving sets around between acts raises dust. To reduce dust in the air, some theaters have sprayed a fine mist of water during scene changes. This, in turn, can dampen the sets and cause the growth of mold. The lifespan of a production may go on for years using these soiled sets. Since theaters often share production, such sets may travel from city to city, carrying allergens with them.

Keep Your Singing Voice Healthy! Anthony F. Jahn and Youngnan Jenny Cho, Oxford University Press.
© Oxford University Press 2024. DOI: 10.1093/9780197629703.003.0009

Case Report

A 52-year-old mezzo presented with a mysterious complaint. She was performing the role of Amneris in Verdi's *Aida* and would become hoarse right after Act Two. The timing of her symptoms was peculiar and could not be explained in terms of the vocal demands of the role. She had no vocal problems at the beginning but after the Grand March invariably developed a loss of voice. Her symptoms would resolve by the next day, only to recur during the next performance. On further questioning, she remembered that as a child, she had an allergy to horses. Since the staging involved the tenor, Radames, arriving on stage riding a horse, the animal's dander was found to trigger an allergic reaction affecting her nose and throat. The problem was solved by taking an appropriate dose of antihistamine one hour before the performance.

Environmental allergies are a particular problem for touring companies. Over the course of their engagement they visit many towns and cities with varying allergens, and accommodations may also vary greatly. Dusty hotel rooms and carpets, as well as pet dander from previous occupants, are a significant possibility. Older theaters, whether on the road or on Broadway, often have modest backstage facilities with unpredictable heating and cooling systems. Several years ago we saw a young off-Broadway singer who performed in a show called *Naked Boys Singing*. After waiting in a small dressing room that was humid, overheated, and full of mold, he took off his clothes and went on a stage that was air conditioned to an uncomfortable degree. No wonder he quickly became ill!

To keep this chapter practical, we will limit our discussion to inhalant allergies. These are the allergens that most affect the vocal tract, with symptoms that fall under the realm of otolaryngology.

100 KEEP YOUR SINGING VOICE HEALTHY!

We will not cover food or contact allergens and will not discuss generalized allergic phenomena, such as anaphylaxis.

What is an **allergy**? The word itself gives a clue. It is an inflammatory response, the body working (-*ergy*, meaning "work") in a way that is misdirected (*allo-*, meaning "different"), inappropriately responding to otherwise harmless agents. Trees, grasses, pollen, dust, animal dander, and many foods and other materials trigger the body to overreact.

With inhalant allergies, that response occurs in the respiratory tract, where the offending agent contacts the mucous membranes. The symptoms begin in the nose with allergic rhinitis and end in the lungs with allergic asthma, with the usual players (sinuses, pharynx, larynx, and trachea) in between.

Specific symptoms depend on which area is affected, but the basic allergic phenomenon is the same. When the allergen lands, inflammation is triggered, with the release of inflammatory substances. The best known of these is **histamine**, but there are several others that are nearly as important. Once released, they cause inflammation, with swelling of the membranes and dilatation of the blood vessels—an overzealous attempt to deal with the invader. The clinical result is edema, excess mucus production, itching, and other symptoms such as sneezing or wheezing.

Inhalant allergies fall into two categories, **seasonal** and **perennial**. Seasonal allergies typically develop in the spring and the fall, in response to tree pollen, grasses, and other flowering plants. Fall allergies, called "hay fever," may be due to leaf mold. Depending on the specific allergen, seasonal allergies may last just a few weeks, or months.

An important consideration is that symptoms develop, and worsen, with repeated exposure. If moving to a new environment, initial exposure may not cause symptoms at first, but over time, repeat stimulation by local flora can trigger allergies.

Perennial allergies are triggered by allergens that are present all year round. Examples include dust, animal dander, dust mites, and mold. These are often worse in the winter, since the air is drier and we spend more time indoors. Many patients have a combination of both.

As laryngologists, our approach to allergy management in singers is guided by two principles. The first is to eliminate or minimize the impact of the allergy on the voice. But we also need to consider the potential effect of treating medications on the voice.

The best management is to eliminate or reduce exposure. For this, you need to know your enemy! This may require allergy testing, which not only identifies specific allergens but also grades the severity of the allergic response. We usually recommend this for severe and perennial allergies that need continuous management. Since year-round allergies may require testing and desensitization injections, we work with our allergist colleagues. On the other hand, many seasonal allergies, especially if they are not severe and brief, can be managed with shorter courses of medications.

Once the allergens are known, you should try to eliminate them from your environment. For example, dust allergy can be minimized by removing heavy drapes and carpets from your home, covering pillows and mattresses, frequent cleaning, and electrostatic air purifiers. Similarly, an allergy to tree pollen can be minimized by changing your jogging schedule to the afternoon—trees pollinate in the morning. On days with high pollen counts, sleep with your windows closed. And don't let your cat sleep on your bed!

After you have reduced the allergens around you, you should minimize actual contact between the allergen and your mucous membranes. Since the principal portal of entry is the nose, we recommend daily nasal washes. In the cold season, we suggest that you use a humidifier in the bedroom—dry air carries allergens more easily into dry nasal passages.

How do allergies affect the singing voice? Apart from the nuisance of a runny nose, itchy eyes, and frequent sneezing, nasal congestion decreases resonance in head voice. Swelling of the mucous membranes in the nose and pharynx alters the bone-conducted perception of sound but decreases the strength and color of the voice.

102   KEEP YOUR SINGING VOICE HEALTHY!

When the mucous membranes become thickened, more sound is absorbed into the walls of the vocal tract and the skull, and the self-perceived sound may actually seem louder. Excessive mucus involves frequent nose blowing and throat clearing. While the vocal folds are usually not directly affected, postnasal drip and irritation of the pharynx trigger cough and frequent throat clearing. Allergic irritation of the lower airways (trachea, bronchi, and lungs) can affect breathing and powering, sustaining, and phrasing.

There are many allergy medications that are readily available, but which is best? To minimize side effects, medical management in singers should be focused on the specific area involved. For example, itchy eyes from allergic conjunctivitis can be managed with eye drops. If the main problem is nasal or sinus symptoms, this can often be controlled using a nasal spray. Since the spray acts locally, it avoids the drying and sedation often associated with systemic medications. The spray is most effective after a shower or saline nasal wash, when the mucous membranes are clean. Local treatment will help with specific symptoms and avoid systemic side effects.

A variety of nasal sprays have been used for allergic rhinitis, and since they all work in different ways, they can be used in combination for a better effect. Here is the menu:

1) **Decongestant sprays,** such as oxymetazoline (Afrin), simply shrink the blood vessels in engorged membranes but do not reduce allergy. They work quickly but temporarily and may lose effectiveness if used repeatedly beyond three days. The nasal lining at this point fails to respond and may develop a rebound effect, swelling rather shrinking in response.

2) **Hyperosmolar nasal sprays,** such as Xlear, draw out excess fluid from the swollen tissues and result in a mechanical reduction of the swelling. As mentioned earlier, using a hypertonic saline solution in your nasal wash also works in this way.

A PRACTICAL APPROACH TO ALLERGIES   103

3) **Cromolyn sodium** (such as Nasalcrom) blocks the release of histamine from inflammatory (mast) cells. This medication should be used preventively, that is, before the onset of symptoms.
4) **Antihistamine nasal sprays** (such as Azelastine) block the effect of histamine that has already been released.
5) **Steroid sprays** (such as Fluticasone) have a general anti-inflammatory effect.

Depending on the severity of the symptoms and the situation, each has a role, both used alone and in combination.

Oral antihistamines remain the mainstay for allergy management. Although a strong antihistamine can dry the vocal tract and impair the voice, there are several brands available over the counter, and many singers tolerate one or another of these with no side effects. Which is best for you is somewhat unpredictable, and we suggest you try different ones, each for about two weeks, to see which gives you the most benefit with the least side effects.

Oral decongestants are another class of drugs that can help with allergy symptoms. The most prevalent oral decongestant is pseudoephedrine (Sudafed), and it is frequently combined with antihistamines. Any allergy pill with "D" added to its name (such as Allegra D or Claritin D) contains both medications.

Antihistamine, decongestant, or both? They work differently. Antihistamines decrease inflammation by blocking the effect of histamine. Decongestants constrict the blood vessels and reduce swelling of tissues. Depending on your symptoms, you may not need both. If you are just congested, use a decongestant—no need for a drying antihistamine. On the other hand, if your allergy causes itching, sneezing, and excessive mucus without significant swelling or nasal blockage, there is no need to add a decongestant to your antihistamine.

Oral antihistamines can dry the vocal tract and may also be sedating. But decongestants also have potential side effects. They may be drying, although less so than antihistamines. They can also cause rapid heartbeat (adding to your performance anxiety) as well as insomnia. So, if you plan to take oral antihistamines (or an antihistamine/decongestant combination) during your allergy season, we recommend that you "audition" several brands and find the one that has the least effect on your voice. Also keep in mind that while some antihistamines are more drying and sedating than others (Benadryl being the strongest), they all have this effect. When a manufacturer advertises a "nonsedating" allergy medication, it usually contains added Sudafed, which counterbalances the sedating effect of the antihistamine, but can increases alertness, nervousness, and insomnia.

Both oral antihistamines and decongestants have a host of other potential side effects, ranging from reduced milk production in lactating mothers to difficulty with urination in men with enlarged prostates. You should discuss any such extenuating circumstance with your doctor and become self-educated if you plan to try these medications on your own.

Our preferred oral allergy medication for singers is montelukast (Singulair). Montelukast is not an antihistamine. Rather, it blocks **leukotriene**, another histamine-like inflammatory substance. Although not as strong as some over-the-counter antihistamines, it is neither drying nor sedating, and has no negative effect on the voice. Montelukast is generally safe (it has been around for years as an effective medication for mild asthma), but it is a prescription drug, and if you plan to try it, you need to discuss dosage and possible side effects with your doctor.

There are also a variety of herbal preparations that have been advocated to reduce allergic symptoms, such as stinging nettle. For seasonal environmental allergies, locally produced organic honey, which gradually exposes you to pollen allergens, has also been tried with some success. Although not all of these have been rigorously vetted by the medical community, they may have the benefit (for singers) of avoiding the need for drying antihistamines or other medications.

10

Visiting the Voice Doctor

As a working singer, it is probably inevitable that you will at some point consult a laryngologist. Your visit can be a reassuring experience or a stressful ordeal. This chapter aims to be a well-intentioned guide, both positive and cautionary, so that you may receive the maximal benefit from your medical visit.

Over the last 20 years, medical care in America has undergone a radical change: despite our best intentions, "business" has taken over what was once a profession. While science and technology continue to greatly advance the treatment of serious or complicated conditions, the management of day-to-day problems has, in our opinion, deteriorated. The pace of clinical practice has increased, with more attention paid to the computer and less to the patient. When visiting some medical offices, you might not even see an actual doctor, and the diagnosis you receive from the "health care provider" can be inaccurate and the treatment scattershot and nonspecific.

This cookie-cutter approach is especially problematic for singers. Singers deserve an accurate diagnosis and personal, individualized treatment that considers the professional needs of the patient, as well as general health concerns.

Earlier we covered a few common complaints, with suggestions for management. There are many others: since healthy singing requires a healthy body (and mind), almost any disorder can impact your ability to perform consistently well. For this reason, we recommend that you find a doctor who understands your craft and is sympathetic to the needs of singers. Even problems that seem trivial to others can affect vocal production and lead to

Keep Your Singing Voice Healthy! Anthony F. Jahn and Youngnan Jenny Cho, Oxford University Press.
© Oxford University Press 2024. DOI: 10.1093/9780197629703.003.0010

compensatory behavior that over time may become harmful. For example, you may be able to sing over a respiratory infection, but to do so you may require a change in support and increased laryngeal muscle tension, which, if persistent, can result in vocal fold swelling.

Your doctor should obtain a full history, covering both your general and vocal health. Written questionnaires are helpful but not a substitute, since an interactive dialogue is more open-ended and can uncover important clues that may not be listed on a printed checklist. The vocal history should consider your training and repertoire, as well as recent and upcoming performances. A detailed discussion will often point to a diagnosis, with physical examination merely confirming what we already suspect.

Although history gives valuable information regarding the circumstances or mechanisms leading to the present problem, **the diagnosis of voice disorders is primarily auditory.** This bears repeating, since both patients and physicians have become overly focused on visual examination of the larynx. While laryngoscopy is essential in revealing visible abnormalities, such findings must always be put in the context of abnormal function. If not utilized properly, visual findings can be distracting and even misleading. With rare exceptions, most vocal fold lesions in singers are benign, and since the two vocal folds look similar in appearance, even small differences become apparent. But if the doctor finds such a difference, you always need to ask yourself this question: **does this finding explain my vocal problem?**

And here is the reason: the vocal folds are often not completely identical in appearance. For example, it is not uncommon, especially in seasoned professional singers, to see a few tiny blood vessels on the upper surface of a vocal fold. If you have been singing for years, the folds may well show such visible signs of use. But are they the problem, or just an incidental finding? Unless there is a clear history that suggests vocal hemorrhage, unless the vessels are large and tortuous or near the vibrating margin of the fold, they may be irrelevant, and removing them will be of no benefit.

On occasion, stroboscopy may show that the folds don't move completely symmetrically. One appears to move more freely or travel a slightly greater distance to meet the other one during phonation. This is not an uncommon finding, and when given the name of "vocal fold weakness" of "paresis," it becomes unduly alarming. But does that explain your voice problem? If the folds move adequately and approximate well, this could just be an incidental and irrelevant observation that does not need treatment. Of course, if they don't close completely and there are other signs of vocal fold weakness, then this may well account for an abnormal voice.

Patients at times get the impression that one vocal fold is "thinner" than the other. This is almost always incorrect. Depending on the angle of how the laryngoscope is inserted, the overhanging false vocal fold may partially obscure our view of the true vocal folds, creating the illusion of a "narrower" and a "wider" vocal fold.

The reason we are giving these examples is to underline the point that **not every visible difference needs treatment.**

The medical management of voice disorders is as much art as science. While the diagnosis you receive is hopefully accurate, it may be colored by your doctor's personal experience, and even a subconscious tendency to favor one diagnosis over others. A verbal description of what is seen on the screen is not the same as a diagnosis that explains why your voice is impaired. Earlier, we suggested that gastric reflux is not always the cause for hoarseness. Neither are allergies. Although such conditions are common, if your voice doesn't improve after an adequate course of appropriate treatment, you need to consider other possibilities, rather than persist. We have both seen singers with a diagnosis of "gastroesophageal reflux disease–related hoarseness" who, on failing to improve on a standard dose of antireflux medications, were simply given double or triple the daily recommended dose with no improvement.

108 KEEP YOUR SINGING VOICE HEALTHY!

Treatment of vocal dysfunction, indeed of any medical problem, can be rendered on different levels. The ideal approach is to identify the **cause** and eliminate it. Less ideal but still effective is a treatment that addresses the **result**, and least satisfactory is treatment that simply ameliorates the **symptom**. As an example, consider vocal fold nodules. Eliminating the cause, excessive vocal trauma, requires a change in technique, with the help of a voice therapist and voice teacher. Treatment of the result may involve voice rest or surgical removal of the nodules, while treatment of the symptom would be repeated prescriptions of steroids to get you through the next performance. And of course, there is a time and a place for each of these methods.

When considering voice problems, remember that the larynx is only one part of the vocal apparatus: it just happens to be the one part of the vocal tract that we can easily examine and analyze. Neither the lungs nor the supraglottic resonators can be visualized and functionally assessed in real time but are unquestionably important. In fact, considering the complexity of a beautiful singing voice, one might even argue that the larynx is not the decisive determinant of how the voice sounds.

And yet, that colorful image of undulating vocal folds on the screen is so seductive to both doctor and patient that there is the potential to overly blame the larynx for vocal problems that may originate elsewhere in the vocal tract. Patients are anxious for a quick fix, and since physicians are trained to fix things, they will naturally focus on abnormalities that appear fixable. Furthermore, as surgeons, we (sometimes incorrectly) tend to look at abnormalities from a mechanical point of view: what needs to be added or removed to restore a normal appearance? Structure and function are not equivalent, and there is a risk of overdiagnosing and overtreating conditions that either are not functionally significant or have not been given enough time to recover on their own.

Most causes of hoarseness in singers are benign and temporary and require only supportive care, such as mucus thinners,

VISITING THE VOICE DOCTOR 109

decongestants, and voice rest. However, even in such cases, accurate diagnosis is important, since it is the diagnosis that dictates treatment. A misdiagnosis, followed by inappropriate treatment, will at best be of no benefit. At worst, it can prolong the illness, and may even lead to longer-term disability.

If the voice does not recover with an appropriate course of supportive care, medical treatment, or therapy, there are several procedures that are available to the laryngologist. These include the use of injections into the vocal folds, lasers, and microsurgery. Before you agree to such more invasive treatments, however, you should consider a few caveats.

Laryngeal surgery is not cosmetic surgery, and the larynx need not look perfect to function adequately. Since even minor surgery may lead to complications that are potentially irreversible, be very clear that your voice will benefit from the proposed treatment. For this reason, we suggest that you get a second (or even third) opinion before undergoing such procedures. You have time: when it comes to the singer's voice, we can think of almost no situation when a surgical procedure is so urgent that it "must be done immediately." Also consider that while medical technology continues to advance, the newest is not automatically better. It may represent a true advance, or it may just be something new that sounds good but hasn't yet stood the test of time.

An example is the current trend to inject vocal folds with medication or with fillers. The medication, usually cortisone, has an anti-inflammatory effect but can cause permanent changes in the vocal fold tissues. Fillers are biocompatible materials deposited into, or adjacent to, the vocal fold to give it more volume or to move the vibrating edge more toward the middle. The indications for injecting fillers include a vocal fold that moves inadequately ("paresis") or vocal folds that have atrophied (lost substance) with age and do not approximate on phonation. While these procedures can be very helpful in strengthening the voice (such as in elderly

110 KEEP YOUR SINGING VOICE HEALTHY!

patients or those with a paralyzed vocal fold), their benefit for professional singers is less clear.

Comprehensive and effective treatment for vocal problems may involve many methods, including voice therapy, medications, dietary modification, acupuncture, and even psychotherapy. If your doctor offers only one treatment option, especially one that involves injection or surgery, consider another opinion.

It bears repeating that many cases of hoarseness are temporary and do not require surgery. If the treatment proposed to you involves a surgical procedure, whether laser, microsurgery, or vocal fold injections, be very sure that

1) other methods of treatment have been adequately tried and failed,
2) the visible findings explain the vocal symptoms in a way that makes sense,
3) correcting them will improve the voice, and
4) you are aware of potential complications and, if unsuccessful, the "next step."

How to choose a laryngologist? In general, there are certain qualities that distinguish a good voice doctor. Apart from being available, caring, and responsive, it is helpful if the doctor is either a musician or knowledgeable regarding music. In this regard, we remember the advice of Dr. Friedrich Brodnitz, a prominent German phoniatrist who practiced in New York and took care of many of the Metropolitan Opera singers in the 1960s. "To understand opera singers," he said, "know the roles." The same idea applies to working with Broadway performers and other vocal professionals. Of course, good doctors know their own craft, but the more they know about yours, the more they can apply their knowledge to your problems. Attending performances, whether a recital, opera, or show, is a good way to get an appreciation of our patients' vocal needs, in their working environment. Of course, if you do require

VISITING THE VOICE DOCTOR 111

surgery, technical skill is paramount, and asking around among other singers can be helpful.

This might be a good time to digress and say a few words about **cosmetic procedures for singers**. As stage performers, singers are naturally concerned about their appearance. While aging is not a disease (although one of our plastic surgery professors referred to it as "facial chronopathy"), it is natural to want to minimize the visible changes brought on by the passing years. And while there are obvious advantages to correcting any visible imperfections and preserving a youthful appearance, excessive or inappropriate cosmetic procedures can have a negative impact on the vocal performer.

Eliminating wrinkles using botulinum toxin (Botox) injections is a common minor procedure. Keep in mind, however, that the performer's face needs to move, both to convey expression and emotion and (in the mouth area) to properly articulate words. Especially on the large operatic stage, these movements are often exaggerated, since facial expression helps to tell the story. Injudicious Botox injections may impair facial mobility for months. Some singers have told us that even a moderate amount of Botox in the most commonly injected "frown" area between the eyebrows has impaired their ability to convincingly perform. Fortunately, the effects are temporary, but for these reasons, Botox should be used in small amounts and selectively.

More permanent, and hence more significant, is the injection of fillers that remain in the tissues. The concern here, apart from a loss of facial flexibility, is the effect on the upper lip. As with facial movements, so also with articulation, the unamplified opera singer on a large stage needs to overproject, and labial consonants (such as "*p*") become more difficult if the upper lip has been stiffened by excessive injection with inert materials.

Two surgical procedures that can particularly impact the voice are cosmetic rhinoplasty (not septoplasty) and facelift. Rhinoplasty often involves reducing the size of the nose. Of course, this may have a positive effect: an Italian contralto with a good sense of humor once told us that since her rhinoplasty she can finally fully open her mouth without her upper lip getting caught under the tip of her nose! But keep in mind that the nasal cavity is the major resonator in the face, and excessively reducing this space can impair both the quality of the sound and the proprioceptive sensation of "the mask." The ideal rhinoplasty should create a symmetrical arching outer appearance with an open and unencumbered internal space: in the words of one of our architect patients, "a Gothic exterior with a Romanesque interior."

Again, with a facelift (and the accompanying neck lift), excessive tightening may reduce facial mobility. Any surgery, no matter how minimally invasive, heals with some deposition of collagen, scar tissue. Overly stretching the skin may impair smooth movement of subcutaneous tissues. While this is usually not a problem, we have seen singers who, after a too aggressive neck lift, complain that they have difficulty raising and lowering the larynx. The key to any cosmetic procedure for singers is moderation: to get a positive aesthetic result without impairing the voice, laryngeal mobility, and expressive facial mimicry.

A few general words about experience are in order. As with learning to sing, learning to treat singers does not come only from reading books: there is also an incremental experiential wisdom that comes from clinical practice alone. Benjamin Franklin famously cautioned his readers to "avoid young doctors and old barbers." While his haircut would suggest that he didn't follow his own advice, it is a point worth considering. The inference that "newer is better" is not always correct, and medicine appears to advance in a linear fashion only in retrospect. In fact, that road to progress is littered with discarded theories, diagnoses, and treatments. Although some incredible advances have been made in many areas of medicine, the management of singers with voice disorders is not exclusively technology driven and continues to rely on many treatments that have stood the test of time, even if they lack the glamor of novelty.

VISITING THE VOICE DOCTOR 113

Do not be persuaded by celebrity endorsements alone. It is based on the premise that famous performers invariably know who the best doctors are. Rather, evaluate the doctor based on her or his knowledge, experience, and attitude. Ask other singers. A good laryngologist should be open to considering different diagnoses and conversant with many treatment options. If most patients are given the same diagnosis and the same treatment, whether medication, therapy, or procedure, this may imply a limitation or personal preference on the part of the doctor.

Also, consider your own attitude. Try not to passively accept medical care but educate yourself and take an active role in getting better. The posture of "I don't want to know, just make me better" may ultimately not be the right one—read, search the internet, and ask questions. Most doctors appreciate the opportunity to explain their thinking and the reason for the treatment they recommend.

The choice, method, and duration of treatment should reflect not only the medical problem but also the demands of the singer's schedule and needs. An impaired singer on the day of performance needs different intervention than one who has days to recover, or even weeks to rehabilitate. In this regard, we have already raised our concerns about excessive and recurrent administrations of cortisone.

What about medical treatment on tour? A performer on the road may not have many options in choosing their physician, so we recommend that every singer have a "home base" arrangement with a laryngologist they are comfortable with. We also advise singers to obtain baseline photos or video images. They should carry an image of their normal larynx with them for comparison and obtain images when seen on the road that they can share with their own doctors back home. In this age of video consultations, a great deal of help can be obtained from your own doctor via the internet. That home connection will help with emergency decisions, regardless of what situation you might find yourself in.

11

Common Disorders of the Larynx

If you are diagnosed with a laryngeal problem, it is natural to turn to the internet. There is a wealth of unfiltered information available online, and Googling is informative but can also be confusing. Many websites are promotional, and web surfing may not give you an accurate perspective of what is common, what is rare, what treatments are standard, and which are more outside the box.

While we encourage gathering information, it is important to start with some basic knowledge that is simple, informative, and unbiased. What are these conditions, how do they come about, how do they affect the voice, and how to manage them? This brief overview will give you a place to start.

Vocal Nodules

Nodules are simply calluses that develop on the edges of the vocal folds, in the middle of the vibrating portion. Since the posterior one-third of the vocal fold does not vibrate (it is rigidly held by the embedded vocal process of the arytenoid cartilage), nodules form at the junction of the anterior one-third and posterior two-thirds of each fold, where the folds vibrate maximally and where they can rub against each other (Figure 11.1). Nodules are an occupational disease of vocal overdoers: they do not occur in shy and retiring "wallflowers."

Nodules begin as temporary localized edema that develops following excessively forceful or prolonged voice use. This accounts

Keep Your Singing Voice Healthy! Anthony F. Jahn and Youngnan Jenny Cho, Oxford University Press.
© Oxford University Press 2024. DOI: 10.1093/9780197629703.003.0011

COMMON DISORDERS OF THE LARYNX 115

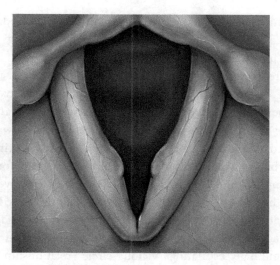

Figure 11.1 Vocal fold nodules. Note that they are symmetrical and present on both vocal folds at the location where the folds rub against each other maximally during phonation. They may be soft or firm, but the symmetry and location confirm the diagnosis.

for the transient hoarseness some vocal performers experience after performing, more commonly in popular or rock genres. Initially these resolve with voice rest; however, repeated voice abuse leads to the deposition of new tissue and a permanent bump. The analogy is to a corn that can form on your toes if you keep wearing tight shoes: it is like a defensive cushion built up by the body to prevent further damage.

How do nodules affect the voice? Since nodules result from excessive vocal effort, the initial sound is that of muscle tension dysphonia (MTD), strained and muscled. Resonance and depth of quality are reduced, and the voice reflects increased pharyngeal tension. Early soft swellings impair quiet singing of high notes: it becomes difficult to gently engage the folds when attempting to sing softly at the top of the range. As air pressure is gradually increased, the vibratory response of the swollen edges

116   KEEP YOUR SINGING VOICE HEALTHY!

is unpredictable. To make these high sounds, increased tension is needed to flatten the swellings, and soft or "floating" sounds become problematic.

With repeated or continued vocal trauma, the swellings undergo a change. Rather than just a persistent swelling of normal vocal fold tissue, new tissue is deposited. This tissue may be soft and compressible or, more frequently, firm and fibrous. Once new tissue is deposited, nodules are more difficult to resolve and over time often become bigger. And here is the reason: nodules begin to form from singing or talking with excessive muscle tension. However, when nodules have developed, the singer needs to squeeze the folds together with ever greater force to try to approximate the folds, which further aggravates the problem. So muscle tension and nodules have a mutually escalating "vicious circle" relationship to each other: excessive muscle tension can cause nodules, but nodules trigger increased squeezing, and so on. To get rid of nodules, both issues must be addressed.

As the nodules grow, vocal attack becomes more and more difficult to initiate, and soft attack becomes impossible. Since the folds are held apart, the sound may be preceded by a soft hiss of exhaled breath, as air escapes between the vocal folds before the note sounds (known as *delayed phonatory onset*). Top notes become inconsistent and eventually disappear. Further, since the nodules divide each fold into two vibrating segments (like stopping a string on a violin), the voice may have a double pitch (diplophonia) as the two segments vibrate simultaneously.

Over time the hoarseness spreads down into lower head and chest voice, and even speech can become hoarse. Remember, vocal nodules are not exclusive to singers and can be generated by faulty and excessive speech as well, hence the older terms of "screamer's nodules" or "preacher's nodules."

Diagnosis requires listening to the voice (as outlined above), as well as looking at the larynx. Unlike other vocal fold lesions, nodules always occur at the same place, the midpoint of the

COMMON DISORDERS OF THE LARYNX   117

vibrating portion of the vocal fold, are present on both sides; and look similar. If the bump is seen at a different location along each fold or there is a significant difference between the two sides, other conditions should be considered.

Initial swellings, also called "prenodules" or "swellings in the node location," can be temporarily managed with vocal rest or steroids. But this is an unsatisfactory, "kicking the can down the road" approach: unless voice use is modified, the swellings will recur. Definitive treatment requires a double-pronged attack, addressing both the nodules and their cause, harmful vocal technique—simply removing them is not the answer. Consider again the corn on the toe and the tight shoe: you can remove the corn, but if you put the same shoe back on, the corn will grow back. Similarly, "putting on" your old voice again after surgery will bring the nodules back. Unless you modify your technique, removing nodules, whether with a laser, surgery, or cortisone, will not permanently resolve the problem. Voice therapy and vocal retraining are essential and the key to long-term cure, although on rare occasions the voice is so impaired that therapy cannot begin until the nodules are removed.

It is generally assumed that nodules have a negative effect on the voice, and this is certainly true for classical genres. We should not end this section, however, without considering singers whose vocal signature, a husky or gravelly voice, is based on an impaired larynx, that is, one with nodules. We have both seen patients, vocalists and voice actors, who have built a career around a "signature voice" that classical singers would consider a liability. For these singers, it is important to consider what their normal "money" voice is, and maintaining that may require keeping those nodules just as they are.

Blood Vessels and Vocal Fold Hemorrhage

Like every other part of the body, the vocal folds have a blood supply. The blood vessels are normally tiny and below the surface,

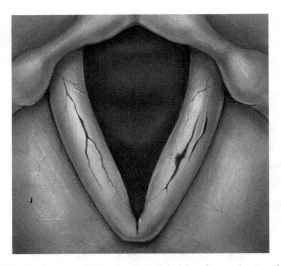

Figure 11.2 Both vocal folds show visible blood vessels. On the left vocal fold, there is an abnormally dilated vessel with thin walls, which may be vulnerable to possible rupture and hemorrhage.

and hence not visible. After strenuous singing the vocal folds may be diffusely pink, and not infrequently a small vessel can become apparent. In some singers, one or two vessels may be generally visible even without vocal effort. These are usually straight and run along the length of the vocal fold but may also be somewhat tortuous, almost like a tiny varicose vein (Figure 11.2). They can also vary in size, caliber, and location. Some are on the upper surface of the fold, others are at the vibrating edge, and yet others, not easily seen, are on the undersurface.

Usually these occasional blood vessels have no effect on the voice; they should be documented and monitored but do not require medical attention. There are, however, two situations where treatment should be considered.

If the blood vessel is at the vibrating margin of the vocal fold, it can affect the voice. Consider what happens to the veins in your

COMMON DISORDERS OF THE LARYNX 119

neck when you bear down: they fill with blood and become bigger and more bulging. Similarly, a vessel on the vibrating margin gets bigger with vocal effort. It changes the mass and the vibratory characteristics of the vocal fold. The resulting effect is that the voice initially sounds normal, but after 15 to 20 minutes of vocalizing, it becomes hoarse. This is, of course, the opposite of what should happen as a singer warms up. When patients present with this complaint, we often ask them to vocalize for a while before examination, so the culprit can show itself.

Not every blood vessel needs to be surgically treated. Figure 11.2 shows the larynx of a professionally successful rock singer. Prominent blood vessels on both vocal folds are the result of years of abusive vocal behavior. However, there is no history of vocal hemorrhage, and her vocal issues are due to excess muscle tension and lack of vocal training. The vessels bear witness to poor vocal behavior but are not the cause of her hoarseness.

A second and more significant problem is vocal fold hemorrhage. In this case, the blood vessel may be anywhere on the vocal fold, but it is fragile and suddenly ruptures with effortful singing.

Vocal fold hemorrhage is like a soft tissue injury anywhere. Trauma causes the tiny vessel to burst, blood spills out into the tissues, and you wind up with a bruise. When a vocal fold vessel ruptures, the drop or two of spilled blood spreads out under the surface of the vocal fold, turning the fold dark blue and a bit swollen, like a bruised arm. The vocal fold also stiffens a little, and the additional weight and stiffness have a dramatic effect on the voice: the singer develops a sudden-onset painless hoarseness. Since the bleeding is within the tissues, however, there is no visible blood to cough or spit out. While "hemorrhage" sounds dramatic, keep in mind that the area affected is tiny and there is no need to call 911! In fact, a less frightening term could be "vocal fold bruise," since the appearance is not unlike a blue bruise or a black eye.

120 KEEP YOUR SINGING VOICE HEALTHY!

Case Report

Our patient, a 38-year-old accomplished jazz singer, was in the middle of her performance when she suddenly noted that her voice dropped in pitch. She was able to modify her singing and finish the set, but noticed afterward that both singing and speaking voice had become hoarse. A few days later, on examination, we found a hemorrhage involving her left vocal fold. She told us that, while the singing was not effortful, she was on her period and taking an anti-inflammatory medication for cramps.

Comments
Even without excessive vocal strain, vocal hemorrhage may occur if there are other predisposing factors.

Why do vocal folds hemorrhage? First, there needs to be a fragile blood vessel, a tiny artery or vein with thin walls, which gives way when there is a sudden rise in blood pressure. Consider again the image of someone exerting themselves, with the veins on the neck standing out. A similar increase of pressure occurs in the vessels of the vocal folds.

Vocal fold hemorrhage doesn't only happen with loud singing or yelling. Any exertion that raises the pressure in the head, such as screaming, coughing, vomiting, and pushing with constipation or even childbirth, can cause a vessel to rupture.

If you generally tend to bruise easily, vocal fold hemorrhage is also more likely. This may also occur during menstruation or when taking aspirin, ibuprofen, or other blood-thinning medications. Keep in mind certain supplements such as fish oil and vitamin E can also increase bleeding. Both may occur when women take such medications for menstrual cramps. However, in the absence

COMMON DISORDERS OF THE LARYNX 121

of a prominent or vulnerable blood vessel, none of these factors are normally significant.

The treatment for vocal fold hemorrhage is simple: first, recognize what happened (sudden and painless worsening in voice quality during or after exertion), and then begin vocal rest. As soon as possible, you should see a laryngologist to confirm the problem, but this is not a medical emergency as long as you rest the voice. With voice rest and monitoring, the bruise gradually resolves, much like the bruise on your arm, turning from dark blue to green, to yellow, and then back to normal white.

One important point though: even when the vocal fold has returned to normal color again, there may be a residual mild swelling that is not visible. Until that residual edema disappears, there will be some persistent hoarseness, which may last another week or so.

Vocal Fold Polyp

A polyp is simply a small bit of redundant soft tissue covered by mucous membrane. Polyps can form in various areas of the body and can be due to many causes. Vocal fold polyps, however, are different. First, they are benign (unlike some polyps in the gastrointestinal tract). Second, they are usually the result of an unrecognized or inadequately managed vocal fold hemorrhage.

The treatment for vocal fold hemorrhage is voice rest, which allows the blood in the tissues to resorb and the swelling to resolve. However, not every vocal hemorrhage is recognized as such! Since the only symptom is a sudden mild to moderate deterioration in voice quality, some singers may just push past and continue singing. After all, who doesn't get hoarse occasionally?

But this is hoarseness that persists, and if vocal exertion continues in the days and weeks after a hemorrhage, the edema in the vocal

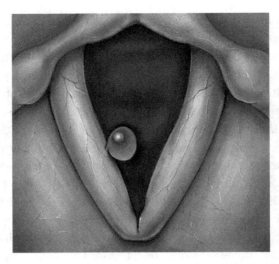

Figure 11.3 A moderate-sized hemorrhagic polyp of the right vocal fold.

fold remains and seems to coalesce at the point of maximal vibration. Yes, that's the same point where nodules form, except that this time, the swelling is only on one side, the side of the hemorrhage. With continued vocal trauma, the local swelling organizes and forms a new and distinct structure, a vocal polyp (Figure 11.3).

Polyps are typically small but rarely may be bigger. While most polyps are usually pale or pink, not uncommonly the polyp remains stained with blood (hemorrhagic polyp). Since polyps are soft, they may flip-flop with phonation, giving the voice a wet, rattling sound that is quite distinct from the dry raspy hoarseness of vocal nodules.

Should polyps be removed? Many resolve without surgery, and a trial of voice rest with prednisone will often make them disappear, especially if they have only been there for a short time. If it becomes chronic, however, this redundant bit of tissue

COMMON DISORDERS OF THE LARYNX   123

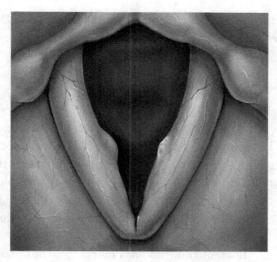

Figure 11.4 A flat right vocal fold polyp, and a smaller swelling on the left vocal fold, which developed due to contact trauma from the polyp. The overall appearance may be confused with vocal nodules.

may need to be removed, since it will continue to impede clear phonation.

Here are some finer points about vocal polyps. Once a polyp has become chronic and firm, there often develops a small swelling on the other side, at the contact point where it collides with the opposite vocal fold. This resembles the appearance of nodules, but the cause is different: nodules develop symmetrically after chronic overuse of the voice, while a polyp occurs on one side only, often after a single traumatic event. Furthermore, closer examination shows that the two apposing "swellings" are different in size and appearance. Figure 11.4 shows a polyp on the right vocal fold, with a slight swelling, a contact reaction, on the left side.

Unlike nodules, polyps do not respond to voice therapy—remember, they were not caused by chronic voice overuse, just a one-time accident. Nonetheless, voice therapy before surgical removal can be beneficial to undo the compensatory MTD a singer may have developed in an effort to push past the problem.

Vocal Fold Cyst

A cyst is like a small bubble under the surface. It is typically filled with fluid or a soft cheesy material. In the larynx, cysts occur in the substance of the vocal fold. They are usually unilateral and often protrude, like a blister, changing the contour of the fold. When they are close to the vibrating margin, the normally straight edge shows a knucklelike deformity. Cysts can be just below the surface or more deeply embedded in the vocal fold.

Cysts are different from nodules or polyps. Unlike polyps or nodules, cysts are not superficial, but within the vocal fold itself (Figure 11.5). The cyst contains a soft material, fluid, or mucus, which is produced by the lining of the cyst. To prevent reaccumulation, all

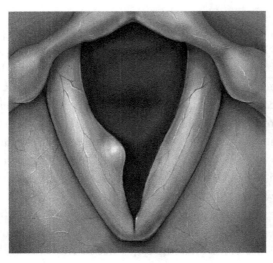

Figure 11.5 Right vocal fold cyst.

the lining should be removed. Depending on how large the cyst is, removal may leave a divotlike defect, changing the contour of the vocal fold, and further treatment, including voice therapy, may be needed to restore a good voice. Quite a different process from snipping off a polyp! For this reason, if you are given the diagnosis of a vocal fold cyst, we recommend additional opinions and that you select a laryngologist who is skilled at such surgery.

Vocal Fold Sulcus

A sulcus is a furrow or groove on the surface of the vocal fold. Like wrinkles elsewhere, these can form for two main reasons. One is a loss of tissue underneath, much like a wrinkle in an older person with weight loss. The other is when the membrane is bound down by scar tissue deep to the surface. A sulcus may develop for no apparent reason or can occur after vocal trauma.

The effect on the voice depends on how the sulcus affects vocal fold shape and mobility. If there is loss of substance, vocal fold approximation may be inadequate, and the voice can be a little breathy. If there is associated scarring and stiffness, the voice may become hoarse. On the other hand, if the wrinkle is just an incidental finding with no impairment of movement or approximation, it may have no effect. The differentiation is made by observing how the vocal fold moves during stroboscopy and analyzing the voice.

A variety of treatments have been suggested, including excising the sulcus or plumping up the furrow with an injected material. If there has been some loss of vocal fold tissue resulting in incomplete approximation during phonation, intensive voice therapy may also help. There are a variety of surgical options also; however, there is no definitive treatment that is guaranteed to both get rid of the sulcus and fully restore the singing voice. For this reason, again, we make the following suggestion: since the singer's larynx is a functional rather than cosmetic structure, the mere visual appearance of a wrinkle or furrow does not mean you need treatment. Be sure that any hoarseness you have can be reasonably ascribed to what you see on the image and try voice therapy before considering any procedure.

Decreased Vocal Fold Movement

Vocal folds usually move identically, whether with breathing or phonation—but not always! As mentioned earlier, we sometimes see small differences between the two sides. During abduction (inhalation), one side might travel farther, opening more widely. Then, as they come together (during phonation), one side might travel farther to meet the other side. The difference between the two is usually minor, but still apparent. The posture and movement of the arytenoids, which control vocal fold movement, may also be visibly different. Since we expect absolute symmetry in appearance and movement, these discrepancies become all the more obvious.

But what does this mean? Well, for some singers it may just be the normal state of affairs! Consider that our "symmetrical" bodies are not truly bilaterally identical: one eye may be stronger, or one foot may be a bit bigger, than its counterpart. And the two sides of the larynx also need not be identical: after all, to phonate, all it needs to do is to bring the two pliable vocal folds into approximation, and it matters little if one fold does more of the work.

Asymmetrical movement might also be due to a recent viral infection that has affected one of the laryngeal nerves. These often recover over time and can be documented with serial examinations. Some doctors treat such cases with antiviral medications or prednisone. Persistent asymmetric movement can also be the result of an older viral injury, but many of these cases show good

COMMON DISORDERS OF THE LARYNX 127

approximation of the folds and no change in the voice. The larynx is remarkably adaptable when it comes to compensating for such injuries, and even in cases where one fold doesn't move at all, the opposite fold can learn to cross the midline and achieve full closure. In fact, one of our patients had a successful career as a wedding singer with only one mobile vocal fold!

We're spending time on this to take the trepidation out of the term "vocal fold paresis." Paresis is an unnecessarily frightening term that is overused by some doctors to describe even slightly decreased movement. This may be an incidental visual observation that has no functional significance. As mentioned earlier, if the folds fully approximate, are pliable (not stiff), and vibrate well, minor differences in movement or excursion may not affect the voice.

However, if the movement of one fold is markedly reduced, or if there is no movement at all (paralysis), then a medical workup is needed, even if the other fold has "taken up the slack." A paralyzed or immobile vocal fold may be a sign of a medical problem that needs to be tracked down.

Other Vocal Fold Lesions

There are many other conditions that may affect the vocal folds and that may require treatment. Examples are papillomas (viral warts) and granulomas (nubbins of inflamed tissue in the posterior part of the larynx), and there are many others. Rather than turn this chapter into a compendium of pathology, we will just make a few general comments.

If the lesion is solitary and not easily explained, it needs to be medically followed. If over time it changes in size or shape or stiffens the vocal fold (visible on stroboscopy) and does not respond to medical management, it may need to be biopsied or removed. If there are multiple lesions on one or both vocal folds, these once again need monitoring and treatment, whether they impair the voice or not. And, of course, if the patient develops a progression of symptoms, whether hoarseness, cough, changes in swallowing, or other problems, medical management becomes mandatory, not optional.

12

Vitamins, Supplements, and Medications

Vitamins are a group of organic compounds that are required in small quantities for growth and nutrition. They are not synthesized in our bodies but are ingested daily in the food we eat, and most people can get all the vitamins they need from a varied and balanced diet. The same is true of minerals, which are needed in trace amounts for healthy metabolism. Neither vitamins nor minerals are "food"; they simply help us to use the foods we eat to maintain good health.

We love to take vitamins! Manufacturers have convinced us that, in addition to our normal diet, additional vitamin supplements are not only good for us but also necessary for good health. Furthermore, so the reasoning goes, if a little bit is good, then more is better. The typical bathroom cabinet is overflowing with vitamins, minerals, cofactors, and the like, most of which our body doesn't need and cannot use. As a result, it has been said that Americans have the most expensive urine in the world.

An argument can certainly be made for daily vitamin supplementation, especially when there is concern that your diet does not provide all the vitamins and minerals you need. This may be the case in those with restricted nutrition, such as some older patients or those on specific diets. The typical daily multivitamin supplement contains a variety of vitamins and minerals in a low dose and is harmless. Additional specific vitamins are useful if you develop a vitamin deficiency. Although dietary vitamin efficiency diseases, such as scurvy (vitamin C deficiency), are uncommon in the West nowadays, some conditions, such as anemia from vitamin B_{12} deficiency, do occur and are cured by taking larger amounts of this vitamin.

When we take large amounts of specific vitamins, our bodies need to dispose of the excess, and this is done in two ways. Vitamins that are **water soluble** (the B vitamins and vitamin C) pass through the kidneys. They usually cause no problems, except for occasional transient dehydration or unless you have kidney stones. However, excess **fat-soluble** vitamins (such vitamins A, D, E, and K) are stored in the liver and can build up to a harmful level. Vitamin toxicity can be a serious problem but one that is easily avoided by not overdosing on these vitamins. Similarly, excessive amounts of supplements such as iron or magnesium can also have side effects, iron causing constipation and magnesium causing diarrhea.

Here are some common-sense suggestions. If you eat a healthy and varied diet and have no underlying health issues (such as malabsorption), you should normally get all the vitamins and minerals from your food. The one exception to this rule is vitamin D (actually not a vitamin but a hormone), which is normally synthesized by the skin in response to sunlight. Given our indoor lives and aversion to unprotected sun exposure, many of us are deficient in this substance. This deficiency can be diagnosed and monitored through blood testing and treated by daily supplementation. But if you are generally concerned that you are not getting enough vitamins and minerals through your food, a daily multivitamin is a reasonable precaution.

We recommend that you not routinely take excessive amounts of any supplement unless for a specific reason. One example is the use of vitamin C to prevent and treat winter colds. High doses of vitamin C (over 1,000 mg per day) may be useful in the prevention of these infections, and commercial supplement compounds that include vitamin C are helpful in reducing the duration and severity of cold symptoms.

VITAMINS, SUPPLEMENTS, AND MEDICATIONS 131

The role of vitamins and minerals in metabolism is supported by almost 200 years of science. By contrast, the benefit of many other supplements rests on less solid ground. Traditional medicine, folklore, and the subjective interpretation of evidence have given rise to a large pharmacopoeia of herbs, extracts, and other supplements, which, although in use for centuries, may or may not be beneficial. Consider further that these substances may have a significant effect on your body, and, in that sense, they are drugs just as much as a prescription medication. It is not within the scope of this book to examine each of these, but we would like to give you some general guidelines.

While many herbal medications (such as ginseng) have a long history of medical benefits, you need to decide whether you need to take these herbs, especially if you are young and healthy. Some herbal medications are used to improve circulation, by either dilating the blood vessels or thinning the blood. This may have a positive effect for an older person with poor circulation but be unnecessary, and potentially harmful, for a young singer with a history of vocal fold hemorrhage. As with vitamins, taking more is not necessarily better, as flooding the system with excessive amounts will not increase the purported positive effects.

The potency of herbal supplements is not uniformly controlled, and the amount of active ingredient in a preparation varies widely. Inert additives may lower the potency of the product. Chemicals used in growing and processing plant material are another consideration. Further, there may be active additives in the final product, which may increase the potency or have an additional effect on the body. For example, some herbal remedies from China used to lower blood pressure have been reportedly "boosted" with the addition of Western blood pressure–controlling medications. If you decide to take herbal supplements, be clear on their potential benefit to you, given your health and profession. As mentioned, some supplements can increase the possibility of bleeding (not only supplements such as vitamin E and fish oil but also foods such as Chinese tree ear

132 KEEP YOUR SINGING VOICE HEALTHY!

mushroom) and may therefore be contraindicated. The internet is flooded with confusing advice, and you may do better to consult a licensed doctor of nutrition or herbal medicine, who can not only prescribe the right supplement but also direct you to a safe source.

Medications and the Singer

It seems that medical visits, almost invariably, result in the prescription of a medication. It would, in fact, be interesting to know how often a patient with a complaint is told that they **don't** need to take anything! As physicians, we have both seen cases where, when we told our patients that no medicine was needed, they went away, only to search for a doctor who would hand them a prescription.

But medicine is not always needed! Many illnesses are minor and transient and resolve on their own. Our bodies are armed to the nines with an arsenal of immunologic and inflammatory weapons, ready to combat many of the daily illnesses that bring a patient to the doctor's office. Furthermore, by challenging the body's defenses, bacteria and viruses actually strengthen our immune resistance and better prepare us for the next invasion. Excessive and inappropriate use of antibiotics not only undermines our body's immune development but also weakens the effect of those antibiotics for the time that they may be needed.

Most upper respiratory infections are viral, and yet patients are often given antibiotics. Antibiotics are not needed unless the viral infection progresses to a bacterial infection (when the clear or white mucus turns yellow or green), and even then, most of these infections, left alone, would get better. Antibiotics are only appropriate when the infection is bacterial and severe or there is a need to shorten the duration of the illness and reduce the symptoms. Keep in mind that antibiotics have only been around for less than 100 years, and our bodies have successfully dealt with bugs for thousands of years.

VITAMINS, SUPPLEMENTS, AND MEDICATIONS   133

Nonetheless, even if an illness is benign and self-limiting, the accompanying symptoms may need medical treatment. The congestion, hoarseness, cough, or excessive mucus that accompanies a respiratory infection may benefit from medication, especially when an audition or performance is imminent. A variety of cough suppressants, decongestants, and mucus thinners are available and should be used while the underlying viral illness is defeated by our immune cells.

There are, however, cases of persistent illness where the presenting symptoms do not clearly point to a specific disease. In such situations, it is important to try to identify the underlying cause, rather than just to ameliorate the symptoms. As the ancient Chinese proverb states: "It is easy to prescribe drugs but difficult to diagnose disease." While managing symptoms gives both the patient and the physician comfort, unless the underlying cause is identified and managed, the problem is not solved. A symptom such as pain is a signpost, and we need to consider that it is pointing to a problem that needs to be addressed.

Medical problems can also be treated on multiple levels. The best treatment is to identify and eliminate the underlying cause. Least effective, at least in terms of treating the cause, is managing the symptoms. One example, cited elsewhere, is the management of vocal fold nodules. The most effective in this scheme is to address the root cause, while the least long-term benefit comes from just managing the symptom of hoarseness from one performance to the next. Most powerful and effective is to attack the problem on multiple levels.

There are, however, circumstances where symptoms need to be managed quickly and effectively, either because the level of impairment or discomfort is severe or because (in singers) there are upcoming singing commitments. This is best done using a **short** course of **local** treatment. An example is nasal congestion before a performance. A decongestant nasal spray will achieve the desired effect without resorting to slower-onset and drying oral antihistamines. On the other hand, definitive management of allergies involves more than just alleviating the symptoms from moment to moment. Similarly, inflammation in the vocal tract, whether from allergies, excessive vocal trauma, or other causes, requires eliminating the cause rather than just reducing the effect with repeated prescriptions of cortisone.

Many general medical conditions need long-term treatment or the use of multiple medications—singers are human, after all. Such diseases include hypertension, gastroesophageal reflux disease, elevated cholesterol, diabetes, and hypothyroidism. There are also a variety of autoimmune disorders that are chronic and require a lifetime of medications. How can you navigate this landscape while taking care of your instrument?

First, you need to weigh the significance of your medical condition: some illnesses simply take priority. Heart disease, cancer, and other potentially fatal conditions need to be addressed first, and you will need to vocally work around these. These diseases may require specific medications, often with no alternatives. But there are many cases where less vocally impacting, alternative treatment options are available. For example, not every case of asthma needs prednisone or a steroid inhaler. Some cases can be managed with montelukast (an oral nonsteroid pill), others with allergy shots, sublingual drops, acupuncture, or environmental modification. The control of hypertension need not involve vocally drying diuretics if other options exist. While prednisone was the mainstay of managing autoimmune disease in the past, there are now many monoclonal antibody–type medications that have no vocal impact. Investigate also whether lifestyle modifications, such as diet, exercise, meditation, etc., can reduce your need for pills. If you need long-term medication for any chronic condition, we suggest that you look up any voice-impacting side effects and discuss these with your doctor and find out whether taking multiple medications may create an interaction that may affect the voice.

Classes of Medications and Their Effects on the Voice

The vocal tract is a composite structure, made up of many types of tissue, including mucous membranes, muscle, blood vessels, cartilage, nerves, and bones (not to speak of its connections to the brain), so it is not surprising that medications taken for unrelated conditions may have an effect on voice quality. Medications can alter voice quality by acting anywhere along the vocal tract, both centrally and peripherally.

When you take medications for specific symptoms, we recommend that you avoid compounds that contain multiple ingredients, some of which you may not need. Over-the-counter "cold" preparations often include medications for fever, cough, congestion, and pain. You may not need all of these, and it is better to treat each symptom specifically.

Antihistamines decrease allergy-triggered swelling by blocking the uptake of histamine. They, however, also can cause dryness of the vocal tract. Since vocal folds need to be moist, a singer may have trouble singing softly at the upper part of the range, usually at and above the second *passaggio*. In this range it is crucial that the surface "cover" of the vocal fold vibrate freely over the underlying vocal ligament; hydration is essential. If the larynx is dry, these top notes will require extra muscular effort or may simply disappear. Antihistamines also have a central sedative effect, which can decrease mental acuity needed for performance.

Decongestants temporarily constrict the blood vessels. When the tissues supplied by these vessels are swollen, as with allergies, the benefit is obvious, especially if you are trying to breathe through your allergic nose. However, they also decrease blood flow to the tissues, decreasing mucus production and causing dryness. The effect is similar to antihistamines, but without central sedation. Oral decongestants, such as pseudoephedrine, have a central stimulating effect and can cause nervousness and insomnia.

136 KEEP YOUR SINGING VOICE HEALTHY!

They are often combined with antihistamines and marketed as a "nonsedating" treatment for colds or allergies. Be aware of this combination: medications with a -D suffix (such as Allegra D or Zyrtec D) contain both drugs, each with its own drying effect.

Diuretics remove fluid from the body. They usually do so by driving salt out through the kidneys. Salt (sodium) is the main ion that controls the amount of water we retain. Diuretics are used to lower blood pressure or get rid of edema. However, reducing fluid in the muscles and soft tissues of the larynx has an adverse effect, increasing phonatory threshold pressure and effort, and decreasing the viscoelasticity of the vocal folds, resulting in impaired voice quality. What can be done to remedy this problem?

Obviously if you have cardiac problems or high blood pressure, treating these is paramount. But your doctor should consider other options. There are several other classes of medications for high blood pressure, and you should ask your doctor if these, rather than diuretics, may be effective. A strict low-sodium diet may allow you to lower your blood pressure. Regular exercise can reduce or even eliminate the need for diuretics as a method of blood pressure control.

If you need blood pressure medication, consider that one class, the angiotensin-converting enzyme inhibitors, can cause a chronic cough that will not respond to the usual cough medications, and such a cough may first develop after several years of taking such medicines. A frequently used example is Lisinopril. The effect of such coughing, apart from repeated trauma to the vocal folds, is increased tightness in the laryngeal muscles, raising the larynx in the neck and interfering with a smooth chest-to-head transition— just like muscle tension dysphonia.

Steroids are a ubiquitous group of medications that we have discussed elsewhere in the book. When used for nonvocal purposes (such as a steroid injection to the shoulder or steroid creams for skin problems), the amount and rate of absorption is small and should have no effect on the voice. However, steroid-containing

VITAMINS, SUPPLEMENTS, AND MEDICATIONS   137

asthma inhalers come in direct contact with the vocal tract and can cause hoarseness. Advair is particularly problematic and should be avoided by singers when there is another option.

Hormones can be taken for a variety of reasons, usually after menopause as replacement therapy. These are usually forms of estrogen, which, among other benefits, also have a positive effect on muscle tone and elasticity in the larynx. Although female hormones (progesterone more than estrogen) can cause some fluid retention, this is normally not a problem when taken in appropriate amounts by older singers. Testosterone, the "male" hormone, is normally secreted in small amounts in the ovary, but increased amounts can masculinize the voice. High voices, such as soubrette sopranos, are especially vulnerable. While most female singers will not take testosterone as such, be aware that androgenic (male) hormones can appear in different guises. Dehydroepiandrosterone (DHEA), a muscle- and energy-building supplement, contains androgen. Also, the synthetic progesterone in some oral contraceptives is broken down in the body to a testosterone analog.

Psychiatric medications comprise many classes and are used to treat anxiety, depression, and more severe forms of psychoses. Rather than go into detail, we will just list some side effects to consider and discuss with your prescribing physician. Antianxiety medications can cause sedation, voice tremor, and hypernasality. Antidepressants have a dehydrating effect on the vocal tract. Antipsychotic drugs can impair muscle tone and general mood and affect. Lithium, used to treat bipolar disorder, can cause tremor and impair articulation.

Dermatologic medications. Accutane (isotretinoin), a highly successful **acne medication**, is an orally taken vitamin A analog. It has yielded spectacular results in patients with severe cases. It reduces glandular secretions—a useful property for the skin but extremely drying for the larynx and the voice.

In summary, be careful when taking any remedies, whether prescription medications or over-the-counter supplements. Do a

138 KEEP YOUR SINGING VOICE HEALTHY!

little research on possible side effects, both vocal and otherwise, and take such remedies in the recommended dose, and no longer than necessary. Explore also alternative treatments for your health problem. We are a pill-taking culture, and many chronic diseases can be prevented, and even reversed, by diet and exercise.

13
Alcohol, Coffee, and Tobacco

When the topics of coffee, alcohol, and tobacco come up, they are often presented to singers in rather absolute terms: Just avoid them! **It's your vice or your voice!**

But is that realistic? The truth is, most of us enjoy alcohol and coffee, and some young people also indulge in tobacco or marijuana products. Since many singers hold down second jobs and spend much of their time in nonvocalist company and social situations, it is unreasonable to demand that they conform to an ascetic lifestyle. So, while we generally recommend avoiding tobacco products and limiting alcohol intake in singers, there is a reasonable middle ground here that you can navigate. It is just a matter of understanding what these products are and how they affect your body, your vocal apparatus, and your voice.

Alcohol (more accurately, ethyl alcohol) is a simple carbohydrate that is derived from sugar. Like sugar, it is broken down and absorbed into the body easily and rapidly, and it represents calories, raises your blood glucose, and triggers insulin release. Mixed drinks often include other sugary components, such as fruit juices, sweetened sodas such as cola, liquors, or simple syrup. Simple syrup, a component of many mixed drinks, is just sugar dissolved in water.

Alcohol has several effects on the body, and you need to understand these to enjoy alcohol without harming the voice. First, of course, is the relaxing, stimulating, and disinhibiting effect on the central nervous system, the reason we drink in social settings. In small doses alcohol acts as a stimulant, while in larger amounts it depresses the central nervous system. This is why, with increasing

Keep Your Singing Voice Healthy! Anthony F. Jahn and Youngnan Jenny Cho, Oxford University Press.
© Oxford University Press 2024. DOI: 10.1093/9780197629703.003.0013

amounts, the boisterous and witty conversationalist may become sleepy, if not "falling down" drunk. When we go to sleep after having drunk too much, the initial deep sleep can turn to wakefulness as alcohol is metabolized and the blood level drops back down from sedative to stimulant levels. The main issue for singers here is to monitor voice use and voice levels while talking over background noise. It is easy, when disinhibited by alcohol, to exceed healthy levels when trying to project over the 90 decibels ambient background noise of a busy bar, rock concert, or sports event.

Alcohol is a diuretic. This effect is due to blocking a hormone that inhibits urination. While increased visits to the bathroom are inconvenient, they are not harmful, as long as you are aware of the potential need for rehydration. Since adequate hydration is one of the keys to healthy singing, we advise that you increase your water intake while enjoying alcohol. Drinking alcoholic drinks when thirsty is particularly tricky since it can potentially lead to more loss of water. This is less of an issue for drinks such as beer that have lower alcohol content than for wine and stronger drinks. Our recommendation for singers is that each martini or mixed drink should be accompanied by a glass of water. This not only prevents dehydration of the mucous membranes but also can prevent hangover headaches the next morning.

Alcohol also acts as an anesthetic, desensitizing not only the mucous membranes lining the vocal tract but also your brain's perception of vocal overexertion. The risk here is again in straining your voice in a noisy social setting and not being aware. All three of these effects work together to increase the possibility of vocal strain as well as trauma to the vocal folds.

We're not suggesting that you avoid all alcoholic drinks: a glass or two of wine shared with good company is one of the pleasures of life. But as a singer, you need to consider the above caveats. Do not drink quickly and excessively. Do not drink hard liquor or mixed drinks to relieve your thirst. Continue to drink water over the course of the evening to prevent dehydration and headaches.

ALCOHOL, COFFEE, AND TOBACCO 141

Finally, be aware of the ambient noise level in the restaurant or bar, and if excessive, do not abuse your voice.

Coffee, like alcohol, is a universal social habit. It is a central nervous system stimulant that for the most part is harmless. We give this little thought, but caffeine, which is also found in tea, is addictive. (Chocolate also contains another stimulant, theobromine, which is, however, gentler and less addictive.) Caffeine alerts the brain, and many have become dependent on their daily coffee habit, whether a morning mug or an afternoon demitasse.

One effect of caffeine that is important for singers is that it makes muscles more reactive. Muscle contraction requires calcium, and caffeine releases calcium into the bloodstream. This is why excessive coffee makes people "twitchy"—muscles need less stimulation to trigger a contraction. This phenomenon also explains the common misconception that caffeine is a diuretic. While drinking coffee will make you run to the bathroom more often, you are not producing more urine. Rather, the bladder muscle, being more sensitive to distention, will signal sooner, and more frequently, that you need to "go." So, while rehydration is important when drinking alcohol, it is not so important with caffeinated drinks. When caffeine is taken in excess, however, it will make the muscles of the larynx more irritable, leading to uncontrolled vocal tremor and difficulties with smooth and soft singing. This, again, pertains to any form of caffeine, whether coffee, nonherbal tea, caffeinated drinks such as Red Bull and cola, or tablets designed to keep you awake while you cram for an exam.

Coffee also increases gastric reflux due to its effect on the gastroesophageal sphincter, the muscular barrier between the stomach and the esophagus. This may be a negative for singers with vocal issues such as laryngeal tension that are associated with gastroesophageal reflux disease. Managing reflux needs to consider reducing coffee intake. A final negative effect is the one caffeine has on sleep. It can cause insomnia, or an alteration in sleep duration, pattern, or quality.

142 KEEP YOUR SINGING VOICE HEALTHY!

Caffeine is a stimulant, and it is habituating. If you decide to eliminate caffeinated drinks from your diet, we recommend that you do so gradually to avoid withdrawal symptoms, mainly a chronic low-grade headache. If you brew your own at home, one way is to start adding decaffeinated coffee to your coffee tin in gradually increasing proportion over a couple of weeks. Decaffeinated coffee, such as from Starbucks, is often not free of caffeine altogether ("hypo-caffeinated" might be a better term) but is a start in the right direction.

The effects of coffee and alcohol vary from one person to another. Some patients can drink several cups of espresso, even in the evening, while others lie awake all night even after one afternoon cup. Similarly, our ability to metabolize alcohol "improves with practice." So, if there are no effects on your singing voice, the above suggestions should be considered as general information only.

Smoking is a different story. Smoking cigarettes involves inhaling nicotine and tar into the lungs. The total surface area of the lungs is estimated to be 640 to 810 square feet (50 to 75 square meters), and the lung membranes are very vascular, so nicotine, along with carbon monoxide, formaldehyde, and other noxious substances, is absorbed directly into the bloodstream. The particulate bits, such as tar, remain in the lungs, and the body tries to get rid of them by moving them up the bronchi and trachea. These particles are so tiny (less than one micrometer) that they don't "drop out" along the way but are carried with the inhaled smoke all the way into the alveoli of the lungs.

And here is another problem: self-cleansing involves the hair cells (cilia) of the airways, which move particles up, to the back of the throat. But nicotine paralyzes these cilia and impairs the ability of the lungs to clean themselves. So cigarettes not only soil the lungs but also interfere with the body's ability to rid itself of potential carcinogens. Nicotine is also a vasoconstrictor and reduces circulation to every part of the body, from the brain to the fingertips.

ALCOHOL, COFFEE, AND TOBACCO   143

Finally, nicotine is addictive, and the cigarette habit is very difficult to break.

The larynx is particularly vulnerable. As smoke is inhaled, some particles of tar are deposited on the vocal folds, causing irritation and, over time, structural changes in the tissue. The vocal folds do not have any cilia and are unable to clean themselves. The circulation to the covering membrane of the vocal fold is also less than to other parts of the vocal tract, so the area is not as readily repaired or defended by circulating cells. Chronic exposure to irritants causes thickening of the vocal folds, impairing the voice. Perhaps as a defense mechanism, the gel in Reinke's space accumulates. This isolates the surface membrane from the underlying vocal ligament and muscle but also stiffens the vocal fold, changing its vibratory properties. The result, called Reinke's edema, is a vocal fold that is irreversibly swollen and polypoid. The area is also exposed to soiled mucus from the lungs and adjacent areas. Over time, the surface membrane can undergo damage that may lead to cancer. The great opera composer Giacomo Puccini, a chain smoker, died of throat cancer.

We spent perhaps too much time discussing the effect of cigarette smoke on the vocal tract for a simple reason, which is to caution you against smoking. While the vocal effects are less obvious in lower voices, the combined effects of nicotine and inhaled tar will eventually have an impact.

A brief word on marijuana. While we don't advise inhaling anything into the airway that is not medically necessary, marijuana may be less harmful than tobacco. If you feel the need to smoke marijuana, consider using a water pipe (bong) or hookah to filter the smoke and reduce the particulate contents of the smoke.

14

Cortisone and the Voice

For many professional singers, provided they have a long and demanding career, cortisone is a fact of life. While at times vocally lifesaving, cortisone can also be a false friend, and if misused, it can cause significant harm. For this reason, a separate chapter is in order, to give you a more nuanced understanding of this powerful medication.

Cortisone is a hormone normally formed by our adrenal glands. Medical cortisone (or steroids) is available under many names, including some you may be familiar with: prednisone, Medrol, methylprednisolone, Kenalog, and Depo-Medrol. Cortisone can be taken by mouth, as an injection, or as an inhaler, and some patients use multiple forms. For skin conditions, it may also be applied topically like cortisone cream for eczema.

Regardless of the formulation, the main effect of cortisone is the reduction of inflammation. Inflammation is a common and natural phenomenon that is more often beneficial than harmful. It is how the body deals with stress, but also how it responds to infection and trauma. Whether fighting microbes or promoting healing after an injury or surgery, inflammation is an essential step toward restoring normal body function. However, some of the body's inflammatory response can also be misdirected, and harmful. Examples of this are allergies, as well as autoimmune diseases (such as psoriasis, arthritis, and thyroiditis), where the body mistakenly attacks itself.

Inflammation often involves some pain and temporary swelling. Again, these manifestations may be beneficial—swelling immobilizes the damaged body part (such as your knee), putting it at rest, and pain cautions you to not traumatize

Keep Your Singing Voice Healthy! Anthony F. Jahn and Youngnan Jenny Cho, Oxford University Press.
© Oxford University Press 2024. DOI: 10.1093/9780197629703.003.0014

CORTISONE AND THE VOICE   145

it further. For singers, the vibrating vocal folds are a potential site for microtrauma, and even if the folds are not significantly injured, the resultant mild and painless swelling can impair the voice. This is where cortisone can be useful. It reduces swelling and quickly restores normal vocal function. Although the best treatment for temporary swelling is vocal rest that may not always be an option that a singer's schedule permits.

When treating vocal fold swelling, singers should use cortisone only occasionally, and where circumstances do not allow normal recovery through vocal rest. However, in the treatment of vocal performers, cortisone is often overused. By disabling the "early warning system" of swelling and pain, it opens the door for further vocal trauma and additional damage. And if cortisone becomes the routine go-to crutch, long-term vocal problems may develop. Additionally, chronic systemic cortisone use can inhibit the immune system, leaving you more vulnerable to infections.

We would now like to give a list of circumstances where cortisone should and should not be used. If there are one or two important engagements that cannot be canceled, and the folds are swollen, a short course of oral or inhaled steroids can be useful. An important recital or audition, a lucrative recording, and an unavoidable contractual commitment are examples. Once an infection has resolved, cortisone can work to more rapidly reduce residual inflammation. Cortisone is also a quick, but usually short-lasting, fix for allergies that can affect the vocal tract. Whenever cortisone is used to reduce swelling, however, it is important to consider what caused the swelling in the first place. Is it an infection, allergies, or trauma? Avoiding or minimizing the cause is better than remedying the effect.

On the other hand, steroids are not the definitive treatment if there is chronic vocal fold swelling, including nodules that remain otherwise unaddressed. You need to give your body some rest, as many swellings can resolve naturally. The correct treatment for performance-associated vocal fold swelling is vocal rest and for nodules is voice therapy. This is a particular problem in musical

146 KEEP YOUR SINGING VOICE HEALTHY!

theater with eight shows a week, especially if there is no cover. Depending on the duration of the run, habitually singing on steroids gives a false sense of normalcy and is a setup for further damage.

Cortisone inhalers, normally used to control asthma, are sometimes used to treat hoarseness. While they may help, they should not be used long term to treat hoarseness. They may be drying and lead to laryngeal yeast infections. If your hoarseness doesn't improve, or worsens, with a steroid inhaler, and especially if you develop additional symptoms of excessive mucus or throat pain, you need to have a laryngoscopy to make sure that a yeast infection didn't develop.

A particularly difficult situation arises when a singer is on the road and sees numerous doctors in different cities. We see this with both traveling opera singers and musical theater tours. The reflexive response to "I have laryngitis and have to perform tonight" is usually cortisone, and multiple administrations over weeks can accumulate in the body. Often, neither the singer nor the well-meaning doctor knows exactly what (and how much) steroids have been given over the previous days and weeks. The goal is just getting the singer through the next performance! We occasionally get calls from singers who are in town for one or two shows and ask not to be examined, just given a cortisone injection at the theater. Since the situation is likely to be repeated a week later in the next city, we consider such "kicking the can down the road" short sighted and irresponsible. So the answer is usually "no" unless we can examine the patient (and the larynx) first and make an appropriate decision. Swelling can be due to oversinging but can also be the result of infection, and the correct treatment for infection is not cortisone.

We advise singers, especially when on the road, to keep track of what medications they have been given, including pills borrowed from other cast members. This is particularly important when an injection is given: the "secret sauce" in most such cases is usually some form of cortisone. Especially on international tours, you need to ask the doctor, **what is in the shot?** If the information is not available, assume that cortisone is part of the magic.

CORTISONE AND THE VOICE 147

Case Report

A 52-year-old rock singer with a busy schedule overstrained his voice and developed hoarseness. He was seen by his primary physician and started on oral prednisone and a steroid inhaler. When the voice didn't improve after two weeks, he was changed to a different steroid inhaler. The hoarseness persisted, and he developed some discomfort in the larynx area.

Examination revealed white patches of yeast covering the vocal folds. He was started on an antifungal oral medication, and his symptoms resolved.

Comments

As a general guideline, if hoarseness doesn't improve after an adequate period of treatment with a medication, the cause should be reconsidered, and a different diagnosis and treatment entertained. This applies not only to this case but also to other situations. If the diagnosis of gastroesophageal reflux disease is made and the voice doesn't improve after a full course of antireflux medications, increasing the same medication may not be effective. Instead, other causes for hoarseness should be investigated.

Cortisone preparations may be short acting or long acting, and both dosage and formulation should be tailored to your needs. Consider the problem at hand: do you just have to get through one performance tomorrow, followed by several days off? Then there is no need for an injection that remains in your body for weeks, and oral medication is more appropriate. An injection of long-acting cortisone is particularly inappropriate, since the singer may feel better but will then crash and revert to his original problem two weeks (and 500 miles) later.

148 KEEP YOUR SINGING VOICE HEALTHY!

Case Report

One of our patients, a 56-year-old operatic bass, developed vocal difficulties while on tour. He had a history of allergies and asthma and had been taking antibiotics and using an asthma inhaler. He was seen by a doctor at the local "voice center" and told that his vocal folds were red and covered with mucus. He was given an injection containing both short-acting and long-acting cortisone. His symptoms did not improve, and he was forced to cancel his performance.

He mailed us images of his larynx. The larynx was red, with thick adherent mucus and a coated tongue. The diagnosis of a yeast infection was made. He was treated with an antifungal medication, and his symptoms improved.

Comments

Both longer-term antibiotics and steroid inhalers can predispose to a yeast infection, an important part of this singer's health history. He was not given a diagnosis for his hoarseness, merely a visual description of his larynx. Not only could he not perform at the time, but also the long-acting cortisone in the injection continued to impair his ability to overcome the yeast infection for a prolonged period. There was no permanent damage to the voice, but several performances had to be needlessly canceled, with loss of work and income.

The indiscriminate use of cortisone is due to several factors. Singers are anxious to get through the next performance, for both professional and financial reasons. The doctor, focused on the urgency of the situation, may not always know what the diagnosis is but is simply treating the symptoms or the appearance of the larynx. Even if the diagnosis is clear, there is not enough time for instant treatment and recovery, and cortisone seems to be the answer.

But the rational management of chronic or recurrent laryngitis, whether due to edema or nodules, is vocal rest and therapy. This may require rearranging your performance schedule, prioritizing important engagements, and eliminating less important ones. Your long-term vocal health is most important, and your career cannot depend on a series of cortisone treatments.

15

Voice Rest

The vocal tract has great potential for recovery. In fact, the entire body possesses many tools for overcoming injuries, repairing damage, and returning to normal function. The Roman physician Galen referred to this as *vis medicatrix naturae*—the healing power of nature. Traditional Chinese medicine is founded on this principle, which is that healing occurs when we support the body and remove any obstacles that stand in the way of self-repair. To allow natural healing, however, requires two steps on our part. First, find and eliminate the suspected cause of the injury, and second, give the body time to recover.

For vocal issues, this means identifying, avoiding, and correcting faulty vocal practices that may lead to laryngeal damage, and then vocal rest to allow for the larynx to recover from trauma. While this second step seems self-explanatory, it is often cut short by busy schedules, lack of self-awareness, or just impatience.

The larynx evolved as a protective valve for the airway, and its use for phonation is a secondary adaptation. Singing, even with proper training and good technique, represents a significant amount of potential wear and tear to the vocal folds, not what the larynx was designed to do. For this reason, voice rest plays an important part in maintaining the integrity and continued function of the larynx.

Voice rest comes in many forms. Complete voice rest means avoiding any form of phonation, whether speaking or singing. This includes the voiced ("stage") whisper and amounts to nothing less than a temporary vow of silence. Since so many activities of normal daily life involve speaking, this is a difficult task and should be used only for specific situations and short periods of time. Modified

Keep Your Singing Voice Healthy! Anthony F. Jahn and Youngnan Jenny Cho, Oxford University Press.
© Oxford University Press 2024. DOI: 10.1093/9780197629703.003.0015

voice rest is more tolerable but also more difficult to define. Should you limit speech to an absolute and essential minimum, whisper, or speak softly, face to face (the "confidential voice")? It depends on the aim of the exercise. Given the widespread availability of personal communication devices, however, both forms of voice rest have become easier than in the past.

Even when your voice is at rest, your larynx never is. It is always moving, with each breath, swallow, and cough. And considering that we normally breathe 12 to 16 times a minute and swallow our food, drink, and saliva frequently, the larynx is in constant motion, even while we sleep. The difference between these normal physiologic movements and the act of speaking and singing, however, is crucial. During breathing, the vocal folds gently sway to and fro but do not touch each other. This is more like a gentle massage than a protracted contraction. Similarly, the movements during swallowing, the larynx rising, moving forward, and the vocal folds contracting to protect the airway, are quick, transient, and followed by a return to a normal resting position.

By contrast, phonation, especially loud and continuous vocal effort, requires the folds to push together for longer periods of time. With singing, the folds come into direct physical contact and are held tightly against each other with some force. The physical trauma to the folds and the prolonged contraction of the muscles during singing are quite different from the normal movements of breathing, swallowing, and even the occasional cough.

Routine Voice Rest

The aftermath of prolonged singing, especially if it is effortful, is fatigue of the internal and external laryngeal muscles and, at times, discomfort. Trauma to the vibrating edges of the vocal folds can result in swelling and inflammation. When we examine a singer's larynx the morning after a performance, we not infrequently see

152   KEEP YOUR SINGING VOICE HEALTHY!

vocal folds that are slightly pink, with mild edema. These are all transient changes that reverse naturally with one or two days of voice rest.

Particularly when a performance is vocally strenuous, it makes sense to rest the voice before and after, to make sure the larynx is in good shape for the show and recovers rapidly after. This is especially important in musicals or popular genres, situations where there are nightly shows, matinees, or several sets in one evening. Under these circumstances we recommend routine voice rest between performances, especially when there are social obligations on the agenda. An opening-night performance at the opera that ends at 11 p.m. may be followed by a dinner or cast party where the singers are expected to attend and converse over background noise. Complete voice rest the following day makes sense, especially if the next performance is two days later. During a run, many of our patients turn down all social engagements, even on their off night. Attention to the ambient sound environment is also recommended, since the larynx contracts in the presence of loud background noise (discussed earlier, under the Lombard effect). For club singers who have multiple sets a night, resting the voice in the dressing room, away from friends and fans, as well as from the loud ambient sounds of the club, is recommended.

While resting the voice before, between, and after performances is generally a good habit, there are circumstances when such rest becomes especially important and may need to be prolonged. In some circumstances the larynx is especially predisposed to injury and may need a longer time to recover. Here are some factors that increase the likelihood of trauma and possible damage. These should be avoided if possible, and if unavoidable, they may require longer and stricter periods of vocal rest:

1) **Inadequate hydration** may leave the vocal fold surface dry, increasing the possibility of contact trauma to the vibrating edges. It can also affect the internal hydration of the vocalis

muscles and require the singer to use more effort to get adequate approximation of the folds, especially in the upper register.

2) **Excessive reflux** such as from eating reflux-triggering foods before a performance, drinking coffee and alcohol (which is also dehydrating), or generally singing with a full stomach.

3) **Excessive social voice use**, before performing, during intermission, or between sets, especially in a noisy environment.

4) **Excessive vocal effort**, which may come from a repertoire that is too high, too long, or generally not comfortable for the singer's voice.

5) **Excessive full voice rehearsals** when they may not be necessary. This is especially a problem in choral singing when singers have difficulty with monitoring their own voice. Every rehearsal has a purpose, and there may be no need to sing with a full voice each time.

6) **Singing when ill**, such as with a cold, allergy, or other conditions that impede free breathing and good support. Singing when premenstrual can also require more vocal effort, since the tissues of the vocal apparatus can be less pliable due to fluid retention. Singing during the period also poses some risks in terms of possible vocal fold bleeding.

7) **Following general anesthesia**, even after short procedures, a few days of voice rest is advised. Whether the anesthesia involved intubation (a ventilating tube placed into the trachea) or laryngeal mask (a small mask placed into the pharynx), there may be some reactive swelling that needs to resolve before resuming normal singing.

A general consideration is that some singers are healthier and more robust when it comes to excessive singing and require less time to recover after a performance. This comes down to overall health as well as the strength, resilience, and reserves of the vocal apparatus.

Prolonged Voice Rest

If the voice does not fully recover after routine "day after" voice rest and vocal difficulties persist for two or three days, we recommend that you first review what happened that was different from other performances. Consider the points made above: do any of these apply? Also, analyze what vocal impairment is. Typically, it is difficulty with high notes, especially when singing softly. It may extend down to the second *passaggio* in more severe cases. If you were singing with excessive effort, the primo *passaggio* may also be impaired. These all represent various degrees of vocal fold swelling and compensatory muscle tension. Rarely, if the hoarseness is more serious, and especially if sudden in onset, vocal fold hemorrhage is possibly the cause.

These are situations that, after medical assessment, may require prolonged periods of voice rest. We recommend initially one week, and then, based on the rate of improvement on laryngoscopy and vocalization, a second or possibly third week. During this time, voice use should be minimal and only as necessary, using a soft and well-supported "confidential voice" in a quiet environment.

Voice rest should be used like medication, in appropriate amounts and for the right reason. There is no rationale for months of silence, since injuries that can heal spontaneously do not take that long to recover. When we hear about singers who take months off to "rest their voice," this usually signifies something more, either vocal surgery or prolonged voice therapy and coaching to fundamentally rework the technique.

Getting Back to Singing

A recurrent theme in this book is the fact that the singing posture is not natural to the larynx but an adaptation that needs to be learned and practiced. Lowering the larynx to elongate the pharyngeal resonating chamber and doing so with minimal muscle

VOICE REST 155

effort and without engaging the tongue and hyoid is a task that is contrary to what the laryngeal apparatus was designed to do. It is no surprise, therefore, that with vocal rest, the larynx will rise and reassume its normal "naïve" position. It moves up in the neck, as the larynx reverts from instrument to respiratory valve. This can begin to occur even after a week, and certainly happens after more prolonged vocal inactivity. If you try to resume your normal singing with no preparation, you may find that the voice is smaller, less resonant, and requires more muscle. If you try the glissando test, you may find that the primo *passaggio* is a bit bumpy, and on palpating your neck, the gap between the top of the thyroid cartilage and the hyoid bone has contracted.

Case Report

A busy and successful tenor contacted us via video chat. He had completed a successful tour, followed by a well-deserved four-week vacation. He recently noticed difficulties in his middle voice. Prior to his return from Europe, he consulted a doctor, who started him on a high dose of prednisone, with no improvement, and he was now three days away from an important upcoming concert. On further questioning, he stated that he had been on complete voice rest for four weeks. The glissando test confirmed that his chest voice and top were working, and his problem was only in middle, with tightness and a "hole" in the *primo passaggio*. He was advised to begin vocalizing and also to gently massage the laryngeal area. He was also told to stop the steroids. Follow-up video visits over the next two days showed significant improvement, and he was able to perform with no difficulties.

Comment

This case illustrates that even in well-trained and experienced singers, prolonged voice rest may result in laryngeal elevation, which needs to be corrected to resume normal singing posture.

It is therefore important, as you "reclaim your voice," that you relearn (although in a much-abbreviated fashion) how to position the larynx. We recommend that you begin vocalizing by focusing on this area, doing soft glissandos across the register shift, initially down (which is easier) and then up. Gently massaging the thyroid cartilage downward and side to side will also help to release the external muscles that elevate the larynx. Once the larynx is back to its trained singing position, you can work on higher head voice, as well as color.

The Vocal Roller Coaster

With voice rest, temporarily swollen folds usually fully return to normal. However, rest also has a limited but positive effect even where there is persistent swelling. In these cases, the acute component of the swelling resolves, but the underlying chronic component persists. We have seen many patients with chronic swelling, even soft nodules, who get better with rest, only to become hoarse again after just one performance.

There are two reasons for this. First, resuming the kind of singing that caused the swellings in the first place will obviously produce the same effect the second time. Also, the abnormal tissue on the vibrating edges is more reactive than normal and with resumed singing will swell more rapidly and severely than adjacent healthy vocal fold tissue.

For this reason, if after returning to full singing you find that the voice quickly deteriorates again, you should have the larynx examined. It suggests that you may have some chronically swollen areas on the vocal folds that did not fully disappear with rest and may require further treatment.

16
Mindful Practice
A Medical Perspective

Over the years we have seen a number of singers who habitually overpractice. They are usually serious and driven students, and often they develop vocal problems—swelling of the vocal folds, at times small nodes, and other signs of excessive muscle engagement, such as elevation of the larynx with excess tension in the area of the larynx above the vocal folds. The voice sounds muscled, the vibrato tight, the singing effortful. The associated contraction of the false vocal folds and ventricles narrows the supraglottic resonating space, reducing the loudness and the ring in the voice. When we ask some of these patients about their practice habits, they proudly tell us that they sing many hours, some up to six or more, every day. And now, they're in trouble.

Case Report

A young student soprano presented to our office with difficulty singing. Her high notes were breathy, she could not access the top of her range, and she felt discomfort in her throat. A visit with another laryngologist confirmed that there was no visible damage to the larynx. On further questioning, she told us that she had been practicing intensely, more than three hours a day for a week, preparing for her graduation recital. Additionally,

Keep Your Singing Voice Healthy! Anthony F. Jahn and Youngnan Jenny Cho, Oxford University Press. © Oxford University Press 2024. DOI: 10.1093/9780197629703.003.0016

158 KEEP YOUR SINGING VOICE HEALTHY!

> that week of excess practicing coincided with the week before her period, when many women retain fluid, which renders the vocal mechanism less responsive. On examination, there was excess muscle tension in the larynx, as well as in the muscles of her neck. She improved dramatically with laryngeal massage.

Practicing has several purposes: first, learning how to sing, developing a basic vocal technique, and gradually pushing the limits as the voice develops, or as specific repertoire might demand; second, learning new music, which is mainly memorization but using a vocal mechanism that is already trained and functional; and finally, developing the ability to sing the repertoire reliably and consistently, which requires both physical endurance and mental strategizing.

To practice optimally, we need to consider what the learning process involves. While there is no doubt that years of practicing and performing bring about physical changes in the body—just palpate the abdomen of any well-trained singer—building singing muscles is not the primary aim of practicing. Learning to sing, like acquiring any other skill, involves modifying the brain. Becoming aware of and gaining conscious control over normally reflexive movements take place in the mind. Mindful control is involved in learning to raise and lower the larynx, integrating sound, proprioception, position sensation, coordinating breath and voice, and the list goes on. These are all abilities that require training of the brain, and not the muscles. As for learning repertoire, this is even more a mental process, but one that combines memory with stamina. So, rather than endless repetition, the key to successful practice lies in the ability to focus, to single-mindedly concentrate.

The larynx is not a muscle that can be simply strengthened as one might do with repetitive exercises at the gym, and a "muscular" larynx (if there were such a thing) would not necessarily be a better larynx. Rather, it is a delicate and composite structure whose function, both respiratory and vocal, depends not so much on strength as on responsiveness and coordination.

The great American pianist Gary Graffman once told us that even at the height of his concertizing career (100 international performances a year) he was still practicing six hours a day. But, the larynx is not a piano, and there is a physical limit to how much mechanical trauma the vocal folds can take. Oversinging, whether in practice or in performance, can damage the larynx, as well as lead to compensatory habits that also impair the voice. So, unlike instrumental practice, which can go on for many hours at a time, vocal practice needs to be better, not more. It has been suggested that the term "talented" should encompass not only a performer's musicality but also his ability to optimally practice. Practice is as much exploration as repetition, seeking the best solution for technical obstacles presented by the music as well as alternate options in case your voice may not be always at its best and you need to work around these difficulties. That "Plan B" is important: we have often heard singers make last-minute adjustments on stage, and that decision is usually "in the moment," and almost reflexive. While you have no control over the length of a Wagner opera, you do over your daily practice. It needn't be long as much as meaningful: you need to extract every bit of gain from every minute of singing and internalize that information to train your central nervous system.

It bears repeating: the brain is where learning occurs. Anatomically and physiologically, this process takes many forms. During practice, central nervous connections are constantly rewired, and potential connections newly activated. There is now experimental evidence (in the developing brains of young animals) that just listening to sounds not only opens novel nervous pathways in the brain but also can actually cause new neurons to grow. Furthermore, these neurons are tonotopic; that is, they are selectively responsive to the specific sound frequency that caused them to form. In adults the brain does not grow new nerve cells,

160   KEEP YOUR SINGING VOICE HEALTHY!

but as newly learned information travels from one area to another (via electric signals and neurotransmitters), previously dormant connections become activated and strengthened.

Practicing is just one part of learning. Learning to sing is a skill acquired through a kind of apprenticeship. Open-minded listening to the teacher, listening to other singers and recordings, and, most importantly, critically listening to your own voice all precede and overlap practicing. Young singers today have an incredible learning resource in YouTube. Never before were so many vocal performances instantly available to a student looking for solutions. While you are finding your own voice, it is invaluable to hear how great singers of the past have dealt with the repertoire—not to copy, but to apply their lessons to your own vocal development.

Memorizing music, like memorizing anything, initially involves electric storage of information, somewhat like a battery stores a charge, and, according to some, eventually the synthesis of proteins, both brain activities. Hearing music and seeing a performance activate mirror neurons in the brain, which prepare you to sing and perform yourself and to vicariously experience the event. So, although singing a long piece or role obviously requires stamina and repetitive run-throughs, real learning is about problem-solving and strategizing. Once a problem is solved, repetition simply locks in that solution to make it reliable, moving it into the subconscious realm of "muscle memory." Optimizing your practice therefore means making use of every repetition, and everything else you do during practice, to stimulate the brain. And this requires constant awareness and attention.

One way to improve your yield from practicing is by developing concentration in other ways. Yoga, meditation, visualization, Qi Gong, and Tai Chi are some of the techniques that you might use to train yourself to focus on specific areas and at the same time to disregard distracting and competing external stimuli and mind-noise.

Ask yourself: What am I trying to achieve from today's practice? Are you learning new music? A great deal of music can be learned

MINDFUL PRACTICE 161

and memorized without singing or playing a single note. Even muscle memory originates in the central nervous system, although not in the conscious cortex. The German pianist Walter Gieseking was renowned for his concentration and could commit music to memory without ever touching the keyboard. He was, so the story goes, able to learn new pieces by just looking at the music and analyzing—all this while sitting on the train, traveling from one concert hall to the next.

On the other hand, if the purpose of your practice is to increase your stamina to get through an entire recital or operatic role, that will obviously require a different sort of practice. Managing vocal effort through awareness of the easier as well as the more difficult bits is part of this kind of practice. Practicing to improve stamina is a matter of managing time and resources, mapping the "landscape" in a way that you know when to exert effort and when to relax. You just need to be clear at the onset of what the purpose is. Like with voice rest, so also with practicing—more is not always better. Certainly, from the medical point of view, several shorter practices a day, each with a clear purpose and separated by periods of relative voice rest and consistent hydration, are better than a single prolonged session of intense vocal effort.

You might test the quality of your practice by playing a little game. Imagine that you were allowed a limited time to practice, say 30 minutes a day. How would you change what you do in order to suck every bit of learning out of your practice during this time? You would set concrete goals, prioritize, and fully engage, physically and mentally, in the moment. Distractions, external and internal, would fade away. The ability to be intensely and consistently "in the moment" will maximally engage your brain and improve the value of your practice.

And the habit of in-the-moment mindfulness, once acquired, can then extend to, and enrich, every aspect of your daily life. A famous Buddhist story tells of a young monk who, after joining a monastery, requests permission to speak with the abbot, a wise old man. Bowing, he asks, "Master, how do I attain enlightenment?" The abbot looks up, points to a broom in the corner of the room, and says, simply, "Sweep the floor."

Mindfulness, being fully aware and in the moment, is the key, whether you're practicing, performing, eating your dinner, or sweeping the floor. Being fully engaged, body and mind, wholly in the present, will not only maximize the benefits you derive from vocal practice but also enlighten everything you do, as a singer and as a sentient human being.

17

Diet and Singing

Our approach to vocal health is based on the precept that a **healthy voice can only come from a healthy body.** The three pillars of general health that support a long and successful career are proper nutrition, exercise, and emotional well-being. Simply put, if you are healthy and happy, you will optimize your musical and technical potential as a vocal performer. While mental issues are beyond the scope of this book, we do have some common-sense suggestions regarding food and exercise.

Diet and Vocal Health

Over the years we have gained some appreciation of how food can impact singers and singing. The discussion and suggestions that follow are focused primarily on how your diet relates to your general health and its manifestations in the voice.

All life is ultimately powered by the sun. We are all little pinwheels rotating with recycled solar energy, and food is how that energy is packaged. Depending on where we are on that chain of energy consumption and exchange, our fuel comes in different forms, whether directly from sunlight (for plants), plants (for herbivorous animals), insects (for birds), animals and fish (for meat eaters), or us (for worms). And our diet is simply what we eat. That's right: "diet" does not mean losing weight on six weeks of cabbage soup or grapefruit; it simply refers to what you eat, whether it is bamboo (for pandas), eucalyptus (for koalas), mosquitos (for bats), or Big Macs (for some humans).

Keep Your Singing Voice Healthy! Anthony F. Jahn and Youngnan Jenny Cho, Oxford University Press.
© Oxford University Press 2024. DOI: 10.1093/9780197629703.003.0017

If you think of your body as a complex machine, say an automobile, it needs a certain amount of fuel to perform its various functions, and as it uses up that fuel the tank needs to be refilled. Like a car, it doesn't need any more fuel than it uses, but unlike a car, it is running all the time. Our cells are burning energy constantly, more when we exercise and less when we sleep, but the motor is constantly running. The minimum daily caloric requirement for a 40-year-old weighing 154 lbs. (70 kilos) is about 1,600 calories. This is what we need just to keep the engine idling. And how you drive your car determines your additional fuel consumption.

Whatever your personal caloric needs are, it has become clear that most of us consume more food than we need. In the US, the daily caloric intake of the average person has gone from 2,880 calories in 1961 to 3,600 calories today, a 24% increase. If we were cars, our gas tanks would be overflowing.

Unlike that car, however, we do have some accessory storage available for excess fuel: our fat cells. We store food (especially carbohydrates) as fat. In ancient times when life was a daily struggle of feast or famine, this was a prudent "rainy day" strategy, but in contemporary Western society most of us have enough food to not need such reserves. Nonetheless, the storage of excess food in our fat cells persists and, in our chronically overeating environment, has become a significant burden on our health.

Fat is stored in fat cells (adipocytes). While new fat cells are added during our childhood, in adulthood they remain relatively stable in number. So, if you gain weight as an adult, it simply means that each cell gets fuller, not that you have generated more fat cells. The implications of childhood obesity are therefore obvious: a fat child has generated more fat cells for the rest of her life, and so has more capability to store fat. For overweight children, potential obesity remains a lifelong issue.

Food is not just generic fuel. Different foods also provide the specific building blocks that repair and rebuild our bodies. Our DNA is the blueprint, but the bricks are made of our breakfast, lunch, and dinner, and continuously rebuilding our body requires a variety of materials. Historically, many cultures have paid greater attention to this important distinction between foods. In traditional Chinese medicine, dietetics forms a major aspect of health maintenance and healing, and many societies today still appreciate (and utilize) the therapeutic benefits of certain foods.

Unfortunately, contemporary Western trends point in the other direction. Eating just about anything is pleasurable, and our taste buds and stomachs don't distinguish between healthy and unhealthy foods. For many, quantity has trumped quality. Hungry or not, we tend to eat by the clock. There is also a social aspect to a meal: we eat and drink as a communal ritual, in the company of our friends. We often don't give food the attention it deserves, eating too fast and while distracted. As a result, we may not eat optimally, with little focus on what we consume, and ignoring our internal cues for satiety.

What are those internal cues, and how have we learned to ignore them? The "appestat," a region in our forebrain, is believed to control our perception of whether we are hungry or sated. This area is in turn stimulated by a chemical messenger from the stomach (ghrelin), which is released when the stomach is empty and shuts off when the stomach is full. A pretty simple switch: empty stomach tells the brain you are hungry; full stomach tells it you are sated. Blood sugar level also plays a role: low blood sugar urges you to eat more. The signal to stop eating comes from a full stomach and higher blood sugar levels.

Unfortunately, our modern eating habits often override these clues. Refined sugars, high-fructose corn syrup, salt, and artificial sweeteners appear to dull the appestat, making it less responsive. Sugars and carbohydrates that are quickly broken down to sugar (foods with a high glycemic index) trigger the release of excessive insulin, which quickly clears the bloodstream of sugar. The result is low blood sugar, which again causes hunger. This is why eating simple carbohydrates (such as sugared cereals, sweet pastries, or pancakes) for breakfast guarantees that you will be hungry again by lunch time. In some cases, the blood sugar may drop to an abnormally low level (reactive hypoglycemia) and cause other symptoms.

Coincidentally, salt and sugar are the two cheapest flavors, hence a darling of food manufacturers and restaurants, so most processed and restaurant foods are oversalted and oversugared. Almost anything can be made "tasty" with this combination, and it sets food makers free to use raw materials that are of lower nutritional quality. The current trend of adding "heat" (such as chili peppers) numbs the taste buds, further decreasing our ability to discriminate between good and bad foods. There is actually a category called "fun food," defined as "foods you love to eat that don't necessarily give you anything back," that is, have no nutritional value. Additionally, when we eat too quickly, we overshoot the signal to stop. As a result, we get up from the table overstuffed and uncomfortable, with that "I can't believe I ate the whole thing" feeling.

The end result? We are overfed but undernourished.

Does dietary fat deserve its villainous reputation? Fat cells originally developed to store excess food in times of plenty, to be made available in times of hunger. They are like tiny batteries that store up energy and release them as needed. And the source of this stored fat is dietary carbohydrates, converted by our liver to fat. Certainly, saturated fats are unhealthy, leading to coronary disease and other health issues, but they are not the main reason that we gain weight. Rather, it is excess carbohydrates that fill our fat cells and lead to obesity.

Weight and the Singer

Body size and shape have always been a thorny issue, and never as much as today, when, like so many other aspects of our existence, they have become politicized. Nonetheless, most agree that good physical health is an important part of a long and productive vocal career, no matter what shape it comes in.

Excessive weight presents both general and specific problems for the singer. The general issues pertain to the increased likelihood of hypertension, heart disease, strokes, and diabetes. For performers, excess weight means greater effort in moving around, particularly a problem in today's more dynamic stagings. The days of sitting around the radio listening to opera have been replaced by high-definition television, and performances are now telecast to viewers around the world, so the visual aspect of a performance has become more important. As more and more accomplished young singers compete for the same roles, appearance, as well as voice, may factor into their success on stage.

Weight Loss and the Voice

The decision to lose weight is a personal one, and the factors that influence it are complex. Weight loss may be medically advised: diabetes and high blood pressure are just two indications. Significant overweight also makes breathing more difficult, increases stress on your back and legs, and can cause reflux, all of which can impair breathing and singing. Sleep apnea often accompanies obesity, causing additional problems.

Each person has an ideal weight, determined by genes, age, and other factors. It is easy to go over this weight, with excess caloric intake, poor choice of foods, and lack of exercise. You can also stay under this weight, but this requires constant dietary vigilance and relentless exercise, and is in most cases not necessary. To begin your journey, then, find out what the ideal weight is for you, given your height, age, and genetic makeup, and make that your goal. It is reasonable, is achievable, and should not have any adverse health effects.

168 KEEP YOUR SINGING VOICE HEALTHY!

Not all fat is bad, and we believe that for singers some fat could actually be beneficial. Fat cells also store estrogen, and it has been suggested that they may cushion the impact of menopause.

Remember that fat is not only stored in the belly. There are fat cells scattered throughout the body. When you gain or lose weight, each adipocyte is affected. Since fat cells are almost everywhere (including the tongue, palate, and pharyngeal walls), they can also affect voice quality. For singers, significant weight loss can affect the resonating cavities above the larynx. The result is not necessarily a negative one, but the voice may change. Once the cushioning effect in the upper vocal tract is gone, proprioception and bone-conducted transmission of sound may also be altered. This means that not only is the voice heard by the audience changed but also the voice that the singer herself monitors may sound different.

A great deal of fat, however, is in the abdomen, not just in the abdominal wall, but also inside, covering the intestines (visceral fat), adding bulk to the abdominal contents. Since singing involves pushing the abdominal contents up, the issue of vocal power and *sostenuto* must be considered. Muscles contract most effectively against resistance. If the abdominal wall muscles are used to a certain amount of load and resistance (like the plunger pushing into the barrel of the syringe) and that resistance has significantly decreased, muscle contraction becomes less effective, and those muscles must also be retrained—they have a new resting position and a different range of excursion.

It is for these last two reasons that rapid weight loss often has a negative impact on the voice. We have seen this in singers who experience precipitous and significant weight loss: the voice gets thinner and loses its lush quality.

Singers rightly worry about loss of vocal support with weight loss. Certainly, rapid or drastic weight loss can cause general weakness with loss of muscle power. But gradual loss of a reasonable amount of weight in a healthy singer should not result in loss of

DIET AND SINGING   169

vocal support if the abdominal muscles have time to adjust. The best way to do this, in our opinion, is by restriction of carbohydrates and portion control.

As mentioned above, muscles get used to a certain resting position and load. With rapid and drastic weight loss, whether through diet or surgery, the mechanism has become less efficient. When this occurs, the singer often attempts to recreate the voice in her memory by increasing muscle tension not only in the abdomen but also in the throat, and an altered, inferior, voice results. The abdominal muscles may need to be tightened and strengthened to regain good support and breath control.

The implications are clear: if you decide to lose weight, include exercise in your regimen. Even with moderate weight loss you need to exercise these muscles, so they can relearn their task during active expiration (i.e., phonation).

There is a small group for whom no amount of portion control or exercise will achieve this goal. These are patients who undergo bariatric surgery—stomach stapling, banding, or other weight-reducing procedures. The main issues we see in this group have to do with the need to adjust the technique (both above and below the larynx) and gastroesophageal reflux disease, refluxing and even regurgitating food. These singers do not have the luxury of progressively accommodating to a gradual weight loss and need to intensively rework their technique. While the issue of support can be overcome, the change of vocal color may persist—with a pharynx, tongue, and palate that have changed in shape and mass, vocal color also changes.

But, considering the benefits to general health (including avoidance of diabetes, heart disease, and arthritis), as well as the increased marketability of an otherwise outstanding singer, the advantages of weight loss for the most part outweigh these vocal changes.

Regarding diet and nutrition, we offer these 10 suggestions for your consideration:

1) **Your diet should emphasize fresh fruits and vegetables,** including those with high protein content (such as nuts, legumes, and mushrooms). Meat and fish need not be your only source of protein.

2) **Minimize sugars and foods with a high glycemic index,** especially for breakfast or on an empty stomach. As mentioned earlier, a breakfast bowl of sugared cereal almost guarantees that you will be hungry again by midmorning and overeat for lunch.

3) **Identify and confront external feeding cues.** If possible, don't eat by the clock, but try to follow your internal signals. Consider foraging or grazing, that is, more frequent smaller meals of nutritious food. Don't let restaurants define your meal size: restaurants often plate too much food to justify their prices. Don't automatically clear your plate; consider taking some food home instead. Also, don't order dessert at the beginning of your meal or immediately after the main course, but give your body a chance to catch up and tell you whether you need more. At home, try serving food on smaller plates; it creates a different visual cue. If still hungry, you can go back for seconds.

4) **Consider retraining your taste buds.** They are remarkably adaptable! Our patients on low-sodium diets tell us that after a week or two of food tasting like cardboard, the lower amount of salt becomes the taste norm, and their former salting habits taste excessive. Similarly, reduce your sugar load, both by modifying recipes (if you cook at home) and by avoiding, or at least sharing, desserts in restaurants. This way you will not feel denied but can gradually reduce your intake of these harmful substances. A side benefit will be increasing gustatory appreciation of the more subtle flavors that are in food and of various added herbs and spices. Sweet, salty, and chili are not your only choices.

DIET AND SINGING 171

5) **Eat slowly and mindfully.** Processing our mal begins in the mouth as we break up our food and mix it with salivary enzymes. Eating quickly and while distracted results in swallowing food that in inadequately prepared for the stomach. It also can overshoot the satiety feedback mechanism that tells us when we have had enough.

6) **Deconstruct your meal.** Separate "quality" from "quantity." Food can be healthy (nutritious) or just filling, and your stomach cannot distinguish between the two. There is an optimal mix of nutrients and an optimal quantity of daily dietary intake, and more is not necessarily better.

7) **Don't do your food shopping when you are hungry** and minimize impulse food shopping. Take a look at what "foods" are displayed as you wait to check out: mostly sweet or salty snacks.

8) **Analyze why you eat.** Are you hungry, or just bored? Are you feeling lonely or depressed? These are issues that you can specifically address, rather than using food, and the visceral pleasure of eating, as a substitute.

9) Since we are creatures of habit, we keep eating mostly the same foods, day in and day out. **Focus on (and improve) the foods you eat regularly,** and don't fret over the occasional slip, whether intentional or unintentional. Eating healthy foods is not an absolute religion, and the occasional lapse does not cancel out the cumulative benefits of your healthy everyday diet.

10) **Dieting is not about losing weight, but about changing your eating habits.** If your goal is simply weight loss, you will consider that your "diet" is over when that goal is reached, and you will likely relapse. Deciding to change your eating habits is a decision you need to make several times every day, until it becomes the new norm.

18

Exercise and Vocal Health

Along with proper food management, exercise is an important part of general and vocal health. Singing is a physical act that involves most of the body. Even if your performance is not overtly athletic, most types of vocal performance require movement, whether stage action or dancing.

We would like to share with you some general comments on exercise, keeping in mind that most singers already have a routine that they find comfortable. If you are a Broadway performer you can probably skip this chapter: whether you came to musical theater as a dancing singer or as a singing dancer, exercise is already a daily part of your routine.

But even operatic interpretations have become more visual, demanding more strength and stamina from the performer. As a society, we have become more visually oriented, and the music industry is following suit. The current trend is for theater directors to reimagine operas in a more action-oriented fashion. The old days of opera as a mostly auditory experience are gone, as productions become more visually sumptuous, almost to the point of distraction. Apart from perhaps oratorios or song recitals, the classical singer needs to move and be physically fit to endure long rehearsals, stand on large and raked or multilevel stages (and navigate cluttered backstages), and keep the performance interesting, both visually and musically.

Not everyone enjoys exercise. Done in isolation, it can seem repetitive and mindless, as well as time-consuming. And in a culture where everything is judged in absolute and superlative terms, the incentive to exercise seems rather modest: it is unlikely that many

Keep Your Singing Voice Healthy! Anthony F. Jahn and Youngnan Jenny Cho, Oxford University Press.
© Oxford University Press 2024. DOI: 10.1093/9780197629703.003.0018

EXERCISE AND VOCAL HEALTH 173

of us will be marathon winners or triathletes. However, the rewards of regular exercise are not measured in medals, but more meaningfully, in terms that are far more impactful: good health, good circulation, a strong immune system, and healthy aging and stress relief.

Exercise has three major benefits: strength, flexibility, and endurance, and these three all impact vocal performance.

Strength refers to muscular power. For singers, the muscles involved in the vocal effort are primarily those of the chest and the abdomen, but the long muscles of the back as well as the muscles of the pelvic floor all contribute to good postural and breath support. While exercising other parts of the body is also beneficial, these areas are most important. Considering that singing involves the entire core: strengthening muscles that maintain tone and posture and contract slowly is more relevant than, say, a large biceps.

A recurring theme of this book is the need to simultaneously contract some muscles while relaxing others. This pertains not only to voice production but also to head and torso alignment and posture. Prolonged contraction of any muscle leads to tension, discomfort, and cramping, so exercising muscles in an intermittent or alternating fashion makes more sense. Muscles that maintain posture are normally held in one position for longer periods of time, with only slight variations in tension, as when one shifts the weight. For this reason, stretching is equally important, and any sequence of exercises should be preceded and followed by stretches that elongate and relax the muscles involved. Stretching also improves flexibility of the joints around which muscle groups insert and stimulates blood flow, which carries oxygen and nutrition. Whether you stretch as part of your exercise or link it to mindfulness through yoga, it is a beneficial part of physical maintenance.

Since singers spend a lot of time on their feet, the lower back is an area of particular stress that needs to be protected. The lumbar area normally curves forward, the lower part of the gentle S shape of the spine. This forward curvature (called lordosis) can be abnormally accentuated by excessive forward tilt of the pelvis, such as

174 KEEP YOUR SINGING VOICE HEALTHY!

with wearing high heels or standing on a raked stage. While these postures are both usually temporary, the increase in lower back tension may, through the phenomenon of reinforcement, tighten the vocal muscles. Being overweight, with an excessive abdominal mass, will also pull the lower back forward, and this forward pull is worse when the muscles of the belly are weak and inadequately support the anterior abdominal wall. These muscles, the rectus abdominis and the lateral obliques, play a vital role in powering the voice, pushing air up the trachea during singing. For this reason, we recommend that exercising focus on this area and includes sit-ups and leg raises.

Although strengthening the muscles of the abdomen and back is useful, it should be done with moderation. One of our patients told us that she stopped Pilates exercises because she found that it excessively tightened the rectus abdominis muscles (in the front). In her experience, since more of the voice support came from the lateral oblique muscles, excessive tightness in the front became a hindrance.

Muscle building is not harmful per se, but with a couple of caveats. Any heavy lifting normally triggers a forced closure of the larynx, the Valsalva maneuver. This traps air in the chest, stiffening the thorax to allow for greater muscular effort. From the vocal point of view, this sudden rise of pressure in the larynx may be harmful. We have seen one singer, a tenor who, while weightlifting to build a more Wagnerian physique, sustained a hemorrhage in the larynx from holding his breath and pushing while lifting. To minimize laryngeal tension and potential trauma, it might be better to exhale while lifting, even if this involves more repetitions with smaller weights. Excessive muscle building in the neck and shoulder area can raise resting muscle tone and predispose to increased laryngeal tension, which can be problematic especially in higher and lighter voices. We also caution against muscle-building supplements. Some, such as dehydroepiandrosterone, include hormonally active substances that may affect the voice, especially in women.

General physical endurance is a key aspect of vocal performance. Apart from vocal demands, the physical effort of stage action needs to be considered. A frequently neglected aspect is the weight of the costumes that a performer may need to carry while singing and moving around. In historically costumed operas this can take the form of heavy embroidered garments. Over the years we have treated several cast members of *The Lion King*, which involves carrying heavy head gear. Apart from the effect of the extra weight on the shoulders and lower back, such apparatus increases shoulder tension and, reflexively, tension in the vocal tract. Moving around may also involve climbing up and down stairs or platforms, often in the poorly lit backstage area, and can make demands on a singer's balance as well as strength.

Which exercise is best? The short answer is, any exercise routine that you find comfortable and that does not have a negative effect on the vocal tract. If you dislike exercise, consider walking. Vigorous walking or swimming exercises most of the body in a general way, and with minimum impact. Walking with trekking poles also exercises the arms and upper body and adds about 20% to your total aerobic effort. If walking is your main aerobic exercise, however, you should try for 12 to 15 miles a week, and ideally fast enough to raise your heart rate to about 120. Most of us don't have enough time for this, so some purposeful walking along with a home floor exercise routine and lighter weights may make more sense, combining flexibility and endurance with strength training. Aerobic exercise, whether walking, running, or using machines, not only improves muscle oxygenation but also enhances lung function, an essential aspect of singing. Consider that, while we all age and our bodies gradually lose strength, a lifelong routine of some regular exercise can delay and lessen the impact of these changes and allow you to continue to perform longer and more effectively.

19

The Living Instrument

The Voice over Time

Singers are musicians, but with one fundamental difference: the larynx is a living instrument. And, while the violin is also activated by the performer's body, for singers the instrument itself is alive, and constantly changing with the years. Not to stretch the analogy too far, but while a violin may improve over the years, the opposite is usually true for the voice. From infancy to old age the human body grows, develops, and then deteriorates, and these changes are also reflected in the vocal tract.

The phonatory purpose of the larynx changes over time. In infants, it basically needs to alert the mother, so short high-frequency cries are in order. The infant's larynx is high in the throat—so high, in fact, that the tip of the epiglottis extends above the edge of the soft palate, into the nasopharynx! This allows the infant to breathe through the nose and suckle and swallow simultaneously. The infant does not have significant supraglottic resonating spaces, and the sinuses are small.

As the child grows, the chest enlarges, and the larynx descends. Since the larynx is still small, the voice remains high pitched but able to make musical sounds, engaging the resonant spaces in the hypopharynx. As the tonsils and adenoids shrink, there is increasing room in the pharynx, and the palate develops more freedom. The sweet treble voice of boy sopranos is the result.

When boys and girls enter their teens, dramatic changes occur. During the growth spurt the body begins to grow, but at a disproportionate rate. Limbs often elongate first, then the body, and

Keep Your Singing Voice Healthy! Anthony F. Jahn and Youngnan Jenny Cho, Oxford University Press.
© Oxford University Press 2024. DOI: 10.1093/9780197629703.003.0019

THE LIVING INSTRUMENT   177

finally, the head. In terms of the vocal apparatus, there is an intermediate point where the larynx is still infantile in proportion but the lungs are approaching adult size. In children, this presents the potential of overdriving a child's larynx with adult lungs, especially of concern in talented but musically unschooled children who try to sing by imitating commercial recordings. Recorded sound is often electronically altered to the point where the final result is not representative of the actual performance and cannot be safely mimicked, even by adults.

Under the influence of sex hormones, the larynx also changes, more dramatically in boys, but also in girls. It grows larger, becomes more protuberant in the neck, and descends, opening the supraglottic resonators. As the thyroid cartilage grows, the vocal folds become longer. The resultant voice change, called mutation, can at times occur suddenly, as the teenage boy's voice drops by a significant interval almost overnight. For a while, the voice can yodel uncontrollably between the old child voice (now called mutational falsetto) and the lower adult voice. For girls, the voice changes more gradually and may continue until the teen reaches vocal adulthood (usually around age 18). The postpubertal voice has become louder, more colorful, and resonant. We can speculate that the larynx now serves a different purpose, no longer calling for mother, but serenading a potential mate.

From young adulthood to maturity is an interesting time for the voice. While the anatomy is fully developed, the voice continues to improve in strength and technical sophistication. The source of this change resides in the brain as much as in the larynx. As mentioned earlier, some singers' voices seem fully formed in their early 20s, while others continue to expand in range and change in color. This is the time when sensitive and insightful guidance and dedicated practice have the greatest impact in terms of discovering and fully realizing the singer's vocal gift.

We grow older, but the rate and degree of aging vary: biologic aging and chronologic aging are not synonymous. Of course,

178   KEEP YOUR SINGING VOICE HEALTHY!

genetics play a role: barring unexpected health hazards, we become our parents! Vocal changes are also impacted by extrinsic factors such as technical proficiency, performance (and rest) schedule, choice of repertoire, coincidental illnesses, harmful dietary and social habits, and general health.

Menopause is a major vocal milestone for women in middle age. The vocal effects of menopause vary greatly, depending on heredity, age of onset, and body type. Absent other factors, the age at menarche and menopause is inherited, and you can get a pretty accurate estimation of when to expect menopause to start by asking your mother about hers. Since estrogen is stored in fat cells, it has been suggested that women who carry a bit more weight may fare better during menopause than those who are excessively slender. Estrogen is important in supporting moisture and pliability of mucous membranes, and menopause, with the drop in hormone levels, can have a negative effect. A sensation of dryness of the mucous membranes is common. The upper notes become less facile and less dynamic. An early sign of vocal aging is a loss of these top notes. They become increasingly effortful and difficult to float and sustain. As neuromuscular precision deteriorates, hitting high notes becomes less dependable, and some singers begin to scoop, starting on a lower note and then sliding up to the correct pitch. While *portamento* can also be a stylistic choice, as it is with string players, such scooping is more often a compensation for loss of accuracy with high notes.

In men, the less dramatic andropause, with a gradual drop in testosterone levels, can result in decreased muscular mass and strength. As the vocal folds lose strength and substance, increased effort is needed to approximate the glottis, and the voice becomes weaker, less nuanced, and more muscled. The glottic "squeeze" often also contracts adjacent muscles in the supraglottic resonating cavities, and the voice may sound thinner and harsher. In cases of significant vocal muscle atrophy, this inadvertent approximation of the false vocal folds can bring them into the path of airflow and

THE LIVING INSTRUMENT   179

cause them to vibrate during phonation. Such raspy false vocal fold phonation has a distinct and recognizable quality, as exemplified by the jazz musician Louis Armstrong.

In both groups, the mucous membrane lining the vocal tract also thins and becomes less moist. The voice may continue to be loud (at a price), but it loses projection and color.

The rate and degree of vocal aging vary greatly. In general, it affects lighter and higher voices more, and for singers who live in the stratosphere, adjustments in technique and repertoire may be necessary sooner than for those with lower voices. Many singers can traverse these changes with impunity by gradually changing their repertoire. In opera, sopranos may switch from light lyric to spinto and dramatic roles, and even to character roles. Some tenors can progress from Mozart or Donizetti to *verismo*, and a fortunate few can even switch to lighter baritone roles. For lower male voices the change may be less obvious, and a bass may be able to continue to sing his earlier repertoire, although with less color and flexibility in the higher range.

For popular genres the adjustment is easier, since there is a large and less exacting repertoire with more options in terms of transposition, orchestration, and stylistic freedom.

Aging is also accompanied by a gradual decrease in pulmonary function. The lungs, the bellows that drive the vocal folds, become less efficient. This is due to a combination of increasing stiffness in the thorax, decreased muscle power in the abdominal wall, and decreased flexibility of the lungs themselves. These changes, manifested by decreased vital capacity, occur even with healthy aging, and would be obviously worse if there is coexistent bronchitis, asthma, or other chronic lung disease. Decreased ability to sustain, support, and power the voice are the result.

As singers grow older, there is also a tendency to lose some fine neuromuscular control. In the voice, this manifests in the vibrato. The vibrato, a finely controlled and symmetrical oscillation around a note, can normally be adjusted in terms of its speed and width.

180 KEEP YOUR SINGING VOICE HEALTHY!

With age, it may become "automatic" (one speed only), wider in range, and irregular, with a loss of its tonal center. The irregular variation in pitch (jitter) is often accompanied by an irregular fluctuation in loudness (shimmer), due to decreased control of air release at the glottis. Since some singers have sung for years with vibrato, they have learned to temporarily cover this gradual deterioration, but it can be uncovered by asking the singer to sing or hold a long and soft tone: the loss of control becomes manifest as a wobble. It is obviously more apparent in straight tone singing, such as early music. One of our patients, an excellent baritone approaching the end of a long and varied career, told us that for a while he was able to work past this problem by singing only *buffo* roles, which involved rapid patter songs rather than long and sustained notes.

While there is no way to completely avoid some of these age-related changes, we have several suggestions that may prolong your ability to stay in good voice. First, as a student, be sensitive to where your developing voice leads, and, as accurately as possible, figure out your vocal comfort zone. This usually involves an experienced teacher and lots of singing, looking at different repertoire. Over the years we have seen many sopranos who are actually mezzos with a high extension and who eventually find their "sweet spot" in the mezzo repertoire. Similarly, we have seen baritones who sing the bass repertoire but really belong in a slightly higher place. There are many reasons for this, starting with just being put in the wrong section in the high school choir! Others include performance opportunities (sopranos get more leads than mezzos), wanting to sing specific roles, financial considerations, and inadequate ongoing sensitivity to where the voice is most comfortable. We write this not as voice teachers (we are not!) but as laryngologists who are concerned about the long-term wear and tear to the instrument.

A particular example of this is the wobble some singers develop, often prematurely, from the excessive muscular effort of singing a heavier repertoire more loudly than their larynx can support. Part of the fault here may lie in putting smaller but beautiful voices into

THE LIVING INSTRUMENT   181

oversized venues, where they need to vocally soar, unamplified, above a full orchestra and fill a huge theater. Not every voice, no matter how expressive and convincing, is up to the task of decades of opera, but the opportunities for other classical genres are limited, and the big stage beckons.

To maintain good lung function, exercise them! Aerobic exercise and yoga are two suggestions. Minimize exposure to pollution, especially in a work environment, where exposure can become repetitive. And, of course, avoid smoking! When one of our patients, a smoker, retorted that Caruso smoked, our answer was "Just imagine how he would have sounded if he hadn't!" Even for those who have never smoked, just living in an urban environment is enough to cause pollutants to deposit in the lungs, so why add to that?

Over the years we have taken care of a few singers (mostly, but not exclusively, men) who continue to perform into their 80s. One feature common to such older singers is that they vary their repertoire and have resisted the temptation to be typecast into one particular type of role. In addition to longer operas, they also perform lieder, oratorios, and spirituals, which keep the voice flexible, and move to these less physically demanding works as their vocal powers wane. In popular genres, the opportunities are even greater: ballads or pop classics are even more forgiving in terms of length, transposition, arrangement, and amplification possibilities. Many great jazz singers have been able to sing successfully beyond an age where operatic singers could not.

20

The Singer

Artist and Artisan

As social beings, we have an inherent need to express ourselves and to communicate, and the arts are instruments of expression and communication. Our sensory impressions and the thoughts and feelings they evoke become real when expressed. Sharing them with others through art not only validates our subjective experience but also imparts a shared meaning to human existence in general.

Singing is such an art, but one that is unique: it differs from other arts in several ways.

Singing is both creative and interpretive. If written music is DNA, that secret code is unlocked and brought to life by the performing artist. More than other art forms, singing (and musical performance in general) connects the past to the present: while interpreting the instructions left behind by an 18th-century composer, the singer is also creating the work anew, using her or his unique voice, experience, and intellect.

Unlike writing or graphic arts, vocal performance is an in-the-moment event, a dynamic and nuanced act that constantly changes. Given the complexity of the task, it stands to reason that no two vocal performances can ever be quite the same. And, from the listener's end also, every performance is different. As the Nobel laureate biologist Gerald Edelman has suggested, the brain changes constantly, and never encounters environmental clues in exactly the same way twice. Listening is an active and participatory process: a song is created simultaneously by the vocalist's throat and the listener's ear.

Keep Your Singing Voice Healthy! Anthony F. Jahn and Youngnan Jenny Cho, Oxford University Press.
© Oxford University Press 2024. DOI: 10.1093/9780197629703.003.0020

THE SINGER   183

Although singing is not a kinetic act per se, there is a definite physical aspect to vocal performance. Sound waves vibrate and resonate, generating sensations in the singer's skull, vocal tract, and chest. Muscles stretch and contract, deep inhalations fill the lungs and distend the rib cage, and air is released in a carefully controlled way, balanced against the dynamic and coordinated gentle resistance of vocal folds.

Further, the music itself infers movement. Words such as "chorus" or "choir" take their origin from the Greek word *khoros*, which actually means "dance." In fact, some languages make no distinction between music and dance. The rhythm or pace of the music evokes a sense of motion, a *crescendo* threatens physical approach, and syncopation is an unexpected and startling stop.

But the truly unique characteristic of vocal art lies in its melding of words and music. As vehicles of communication, words are digital, and music is analog. Words are discrete bits of data that, even when poetic and evocative, speak primarily to the rational and analytic left brain. Music, on the other hand, speaks to the right brain, the brain that is instinctive, intuitive, and emotional. As the soprano Christine Goerke insightfully observed, in an operatic aria words may convey meaning, but it is the music that conveys intent. And it is this yoking together of words and music, of meaning and intent, that makes singing unique among all other forms of arts. Basso Luca Pisaroni put it simply: "Singing lets me say things I cannot say with words."

"Art" has transcendent connotations, but there is another, lower case, definition of art, which is **art as craft**. Craft is the servant of Art, and the artist is also an artisan. Vocal performance requires technical mastery, and it is craft that separates the longing amateur from the competent professional. And, although "Art" refers to expression on a higher plane, this older, and more prosaic, definition remains embedded in its meaning. In this sense, the term shares its origins with "artificial" and "artifice." After all, the "Artful Dodger" in Dickens's *Oliver Twist* was nothing but a sly and skillful pickpocket!

184 KEEP YOUR SINGING VOICE HEALTHY!

Ultimately all art is illusion, whether a painted landscape seeming to recede to a vanishing point, the frozen-in-time "movement" of a sculpture, or the emotional urgency of a song. The mastery of art is to convincingly present that illusion for the observer or listener, to be adept at evocative deception. And to create that convincing illusion, the true artist must first be skilled. The pianist Yefim Bronfman stated it prosaically: interpretation is important, but you also must hit the right notes! As masterful deceiver, the artist's goal is to convince us by making the artificial seem effortless and natural. *Ars est celare Artem*: the art is to hide art. In the case of singers, this requires a thorough understanding and control of that dynamic and ever-changing instrument that is their own body.

But once the *artisan* masters her or his craft, that key opens the door for the *Artist*: the performer, who follows the composer's instructions, becomes the interpreter, and conveys the composer's intent and meaning. And the result, the song, the melding of craft and art, is both very personal and immensely universal, a truly unique Art that is like no other.

APPENDIX 1

Ten Simple Tips for Keeping Your Voice Healthy

1. Speak like you sing, with good technique.

2. Stay hydrated. Drink eight-oz. glasses of water every day—two glasses of water with each meal and one glass between meals $(2 + 1 + 2 + 1 + 2 = 8)$.

3. Know your body. When you are ill, don't force the voice.

4. If it hurts to sing, stop and reassess. You're doing something wrong.

5. Avoid noisy places if you can. Even if you are not speaking, your throat tenses reflexively.

6. For an optimal diet, eat small amounts of healthy food frequently.

7. Identify, and deal with, harmful stressors in your life.

8. Address muscle tension anywhere in your body. It can heighten tension in your vocal tract.

9. Exercise and stretch regularly.

10. Be aware of your medications (prescription, over the counter, and supplements), including possible effects on the voice.

APPENDIX 2

Anatomic Intermezzo
What Do You Call That Thing?

As medical words have increasingly become part of the singers' academic curriculum, singers are faced with memorizing the names of parts of the vocal tract, a rather dry task!

To lighten the burden, we thought you might enjoy looking at the origins of some of these names. Many have an ancient and evocative history, and they often come from a time before modern medicine understood their true structure and function. But the names persist, and they resonate with the history and romance of anatomy.

Some structures are simply named after the objects they resemble. The **uvula** is a good example.

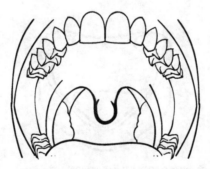

The uvula has an ovoid, rounded shape, like a small grape.

This small appendage hangs from the free margin of the soft palate. It acts as a dripspout that collects nasal secretions from the upper surface of the palate and allows them to drip to the back of the tongue. Although we have heard patients prosaically refer to the uvula as "the punching bag," the original name is more poetic: it means a small grape (*uva* being Latin for "grape").

But the uvula is not the only fruit in the neighborhood! In many languages the **tonsils** are called "almonds" (e.g., *Mandeln* in German), due to their shape and pitted appearance, and the food gutters on either side of the larynx are the **pyriform fossae**, the pear-shaped trenches.

The names of the three main cartilages of the larynx paint an image from daily life in ancient times: the **thyroid cartilage** resembles a foot soldier's shield, the **cricoid cartilage** looks like a signet ring, and the **arytenoid cartilage** recalls the shape of a water jug or ewer.

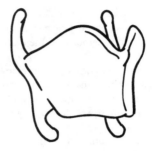

The thyroid cartilage is reminiscent of the large shield carried by Roman foot soldiers.

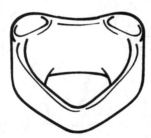

The cricoid cartilage looks somewhat like a signet ring.

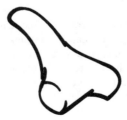

The arytenoid cartilage is shaped like a ewer, or water jug.

APPENDIX 2   189

Some references are prosaic, while others can at times be quite fanciful. The **hyoid bone** is named after the Greek letter upsilon, since in resembles an upside-down letter "U." While the term "**palate**" for the roof of the mouth is in common use, surgical books of the late 1800s referred to palate surgery not as "palatoplasty" but as "uranoplasty." The reference was to Uranus, ancient Greek god of the sky and grandfather of Zeus. The metaphor likens the palate to the celestial vault, arching above the earth. And those large round **taste buds** on the back of the tongue (did you ever wonder what those big bumps were?) are called the **circumvallate papillae**, the term suggesting small medieval towers surrounded by a moat or trench (circumvallum).

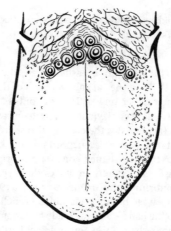

The circumvallate tastebuds on the back of the tongue look like a line of small round forts, surrounded by moats.

Now obsolete, many older names simply reflected an ignorance of function. For example, the **trachea** was originally called *arteria aspera*, or "rough artery." To Renaissance anatomists secretly dissecting cadavers by torchlight, the trachea may indeed have resembled a large hollow artery with corrugated walls.

Muscles are often named after the structures to which they attach. The **sternocleidomastoid** (SCM) muscle, the main straplike muscle that runs obliquely across each side of the neck, is responsible for turning the head.

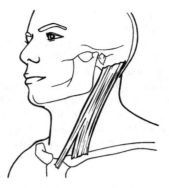

The sternocleidomastoid muscle takes its name from its attachments: the mastoid process behind the ear, and the clavicle and sternum below.

The SCM connects the **sternum** (breastbone) and the **clavicle**, below, with the **mastoid** process (behind the ear) above. Each of these bony structures, in turn, evokes a much richer image. The mastoid is "breast shaped." The clavicle resembles a small key (claviculum), perhaps a wrought-iron key to an ancient dungeon. Incidentally, the clavicle also shares its derivation with keyboard instruments such as the clavichord and the klavier, as well as the Cuban claves. Perhaps this key-shaped bone was the original "skeleton key"?

However, the breastbone, or sternum, takes the etymologic cake! Its two main parts, the **manubrium** (the smaller upper part that articulates with the clavicles) and the larger body, or **gladiolus** (which articulates with the ribs), refer, in turn, to the handle and the blade of a short Roman sword. Men wielding this breastbone-shaped weapon in lethal battle came to be known as the gladiators. The gladiator, with his short sword and shield, was pitted against another fighter, who was armed with a trident and a net, in a fight to the death. And you thought singing was difficult?

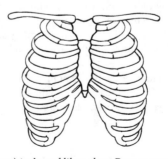

The breastbone (sternum) is shaped like a short Roman sword.

APPENDIX 2   191

Yet other names commemorate great doctors otherwise forgotten. The Eustachian tubes allude to Bartolomeo Eustachi, a renowned anatomist from Renaissance Padua, one of the first medical schools that permitted the dissection of dead bodies. And the two tiny accessory cartilages of the larynx (don't worry if you don't know these: they are really small, and of no significance to singers) are both descriptive and allusive: they are the corniculate ("like a little horn") and cuneiform ("wedge shaped") cartilages, but also perpetuate the memory of the anatomists Santorini and Wirsung.

There even seems to be a nationalistic edge to the medical name game: a single condition, chronic autoimmune inflammation of the thyroid gland, can be referred to as either Graves's disease, Basedow's disease, or Hashimoto's thyroiditis, depending on whether you are English, Russian, or Japanese!

Even today we continue to rename structures, to reflect our growing understanding of their true structure or function. Perhaps most illustrative for singers is the renaming of the two vibrating structures that produce the voice. The older term "**vocal cords**" implied two taut strings. While to the gross anatomist looking at a dry specimen this may be a valid description, it does not reflect the structural complexity of these structures, and the fact that they are covered by a somewhat loose surface epithelium. "**Vocal folds**" has therefore become the currently accepted term.

Yet, neither term tells the entire story. While "vocal cord" might describe the vocal ligament, and "vocal fold" the overlying epithelium ("fold" implies a bunching up or redundancy of a single layer, such as a fold in a piece of cloth), neither term speaks to its function. So the definitive name (at least in English) is still waiting to be invented. The best current descriptive term may well be the German *Stimmlippen* or "voice lips": the word describes what these structures do, rather than just their appearance, and the comparison to the multilayered and sphincterlike lips implies a complexity that both "vocal cords" and "vocal folds" miss.

Index

For the benefit of digital users, indexed terms that span two pages (e.g., 52–53) may, on occasion, appear on only one of those pages.

Tables, figures, and boxes are indicated by an italic *t*, *f*, and *b* following the page/paragraph number.

abdominal breathing
  exhalation phase, 2
  hypodermic syringe comparison, 4
  inhalation phase, 2
  mechanisms of inhalation/exhalation,
    2–4, 3*f*
  role of the diaphragm, abdominal
    muscles, 2–4
  singing naturally *vs.* trained singing,
    22*t*
abdominal muscles, 1, 2–4, 6, 168–69
acid reflux, 90–94
  constant throat clearing and, 77
  gastroesophageal disease and, 91–94
  management of, 93
  pharyngeal irritation from, 77
  reflux, defined, 91
  reflux-induced laryngeal tension from,
    93
  secondary laryngeal tension and,
    66–67
  voice damage from, 92–93
  See also gastroesophageal
    disease (GERD)
acupuncture, 90, 110, 134
aging voice. *See* voice changes over time
agonist-antagonist muscles, 8, 51, 52
air conduction, 37–38, 38*f*, 40, 45–47
alcohol
  anesthetic effect, 140
  comparison to coffee, 142
  dehydrating effect of, 78–79
  diuretic effect of, 140

  reflux, GERD, and, 92, 96
  stimulating/depressive effects, 139–40
  suggestions for singers, 140–41
  varied effects of, 142
allergic rhinitis, 100, 102
allergies, 98–104
  allergy, defined, 100
  case report, hoarseness, 99*b*
  environmental allergies, 99
  food allergies, 77
  impact on the singing voice, 101–2
  inhalant allergies, 76, 79–80, 100
  nasal allergies/sinusitis, 79, 85–86
  perennial/seasonal allargies, 100–1
  proneness of singers to, 98
  specific symptoms, 100
  triggering of histamine, 100
  See also allergies, management
allergies, management, 101, 102–3
  antihistamine nasal sprays, 103
  cromolyn sodium, 103
  decongestant sprays, 102
  hyperosmolar nasal sprays, 102
  monteleukast, as preferred for singers,
    104, 134
  oral antihistamines, 103–4
  oral decongestants, 87, 103, 135–36
  potential medication side effects, 104
  steroid sprays, 103
antihistamines
  case report/for hoarseness, 99*b*
  consequences of inapproriate use, 78
  decongestants comparison, 135–36

194 INDEX

antihistamines (*cont.*)
 description, 103
 Monteleukast comparison, 104
 nasal sprays, 103
 oral, 103–4, 133–34
 potential side effects of, 104, 135
appoggio, defined, 6–7
auditory fatigue, 26

belting
 safe belting techniques, 25
 In transition from chest to head voice, 25
blood vessels, vocal fold hemorrhage, 117–21, 118*f*
bone conduction, 37–39, 38*f*, 45, 46–47
bruxism (clenching, grinding), 61–64, 63*f*
 causes of, 64
 checking for, 62
 impact on the TMJs, 62

chest voice
 anatomy of, 23*f*
 belting and, 25
 "chest register" muscles and, 24
 defined, 33–34
 hoarseness and, 116
 mezzos and, 27
 role of laryngeal muscles, 23
 transition to head voice, 24–25, 33–34, 42
cigarette smoking
 description/negative effects, 142–43
 impact on the larynx, 143
coffee
 caffeine's stimulating effect, 141
 comparison to alcohol, 142
 habituating effect, 142
 impact on muscles, 141
 reflux, GERD, and, 92, 141
 varied effects of, 142
compensation-related muscle tension, 65
complaints
 acid reflux, 90
 case report: loss of voice, 67*b*
 consideration of context, 74

headache, 85–86, 94
hoarseness, 95
mucus, 75–80
nasal obstruction, 83
post-singing throat discomfort, 88
sinusitis, 85
throat infections, 76
tonsillitis, 82
vocal strain, management, 89
"the voice doesn't feel right," 41
cortisone (medical cortisone), 144–46, 147–48*b*
 case report/hoarseness, 147*b*
 case report/vocal fold irritation, 148*b*
 description, 144
 effects of, 144
 factors in determining use of, 145–46
 injections, 66, 136–37, 144, 146, 148*b*
 long-term use risks, 145
 oral/inhaled, 145, 147, 147b, 148b
 reasons for indiscriminate use of, 148
 short *vs.* long acting preparations, 147
 for vocal fold swelling, 145
cosmetic procedures for singers, 111–12
 botulinum toxin (Botox) injections, 111
 cosmetic rhinoplasty/facelift, 111–12
 injection of fillers, 111
cough
 acid reflux and, 94
 allergies and, 101–2
 excess mucus and, 76
 hoarseness and, 42
 importance of, 6
 medications for, 133, 135
 as medication side-effect, 136
 triggers of, 6
 vocal fold hemorrhage and, 119, 120
 vocal fold lesions and, 127–28
 vocal hemorrhage and, 96–97
cricothyroid muscles, 23*f*, 24, 33–34
cromolyn sodium, 103

decongestants
 mechanisms of action, 103, 135–36
 nasal sprays, 6–7, 85, 86–88
 oral, 87, 103, 135–36

INDEX 195

for persistent illness, 133
potential side effects, 103–4
topical sprays, 86, 94, 102
use in neti pot, 86
dermatologic medications, 137–38
diaphragm
role in abdominal breathing, 2–4, 3f
singing from the diaphragm, 2
diet and nutrition, 163–71
caffeine and, 142
daily caloric requirement, 164
defined, 163
dietary considerations, 169–71
dietary fat, 164, 166, 168
downside of modern eating habits, 165–66
exercise and, 172
four-week elimination, 80
lifestyle modifications and, 134
low-sodium, 136
reflux management and, 93
vitamin supplements and, 129–30
vocal health and, 163–66
weight considerations, 166–71
weight loss and, 93
See also vitamins and
minerals; weight
diuretic medication, 136

ears
anatomy of, 45–46, 46f
cross-sectional diagram, 46f
inner ear, 26
path of sound to, 37–38, 38f, 41–45
sound sensitivity of, 48
stimulus for listening, 9–10
warble tone stimulus, 26
ethnic singing, 21–22
exercise, 172–75
abdomen and lower back, 173–74
avoidance, for vocal strain, 89
benefits for blood pressure, 136
benefits of, 137–38, 173
choices/types of, 175
hydration and, 78–79
muscle building, 174
physical endurance, 175

pills *vs.*, 137–38
vocal health and, 172–75
voice rest and, 150–51
weight loss and, 167, 169

fach, vocal range and, 27, 28–29, 30
false vocal folds, 5, 15, 53–54,
157, 178–79

Galen (Roman physician), 150
Garcia, Manuel, 35
gastroesophageal disease (GERD)
excessive mucus/throat clearing and, 92
hypopharynx, throat pain, and, 91
management of, 92, 93
muscle tension dysphonia comparison, 93
night *vs.* morning throat pain, 91
reflux and, 91–94
self-diagnosis/treatment, 91–92
See also acid reflux
glissando, vocal folds and, 23–24
glissando test, 41–44
case report/middle voice tightness,
155b
description, 42
evaluation of, 42
focus on *primo passaggio,* 42–43
focus on *secondo passaggio,* 43
for hoarseness, strain, 42, 88, 96
reasons for impaired transition points,
43–44

headache, 85–86, 94
bruxism, TMJ, and, 94–95
determination of cause, 94
determination of location, 94–95
sinusitis and, 94
vacuum headache phenomenon, 85–86
head voice
belting and, 25
chest voice transition to, 24–25, 33–
34, 42
distinction from chest voice, 23
glissando test for hoarseness in, 88
impact of allergies, 101–2

196 INDEX

head voice (*cont.*)
  muscle tension and, 53, 58*b*
  role of laryngeal muscles, 23*f*, 23
  term derivation, 85
  vocal fold and, 10*f*
  women and, 29–30
hearing
  air conduction/bone conduction and, 45–47
  conductive portion, 45, 47
  impact of noise pollution, 48–49
  importance for singing, 45
  Lombard effect and, 49, 152
  mechanics of, 45
  role in gauging loudness and pitch, 47
  sensory portion, 45, 47
  singer's ears monitoring of, 46–47
  singing and, 45–50
  tinnitus and, 48, 49–50
  See also ears; hearing loss
hearing loss
  acute (sudden) onset, 47
  audiology testing for, 22–23
  conductive *vs.* sensory, 47
  early signs of, 48
  gradual, 47–48
  industrial loudness standards, 48–49
  mixed, 45
  signs of, 48
  singing with impaired hearing, 22–23
  strategies for preventing, 48–49
  sudden *vs.* gradual loss, 47–48
  tinnitus and, 48, 49–50
Helmholtz, Hermann, 12–13, 13*f*
herbal medications, 131–32
hoarseness, 95–97
  case report, chronic hoarseness, 71*b*
  chest voice and, 116
  description, 95–96
  glissando test for, 42, 88, 96
  laryngologist diagnosis, 97
  laryngologist treatments, 110
  medications for, 133
  oversinging and, 90
  primary causes of, 108–9
  reflux/GERD and morning hoarseness, 92, 93–94

secondo passaggio and, 43
virus infection and, 97
vocal fold polyp and, 121–22
vocal nodules and, 116
voice rest for, 97, 108–9
hormone treatments, 137
humidifiers, 79–80, 83–84, 101
hyperosmolar nasal sprays, 102
hypertension (high blood pressure), 136, 167
hypopharynx
  engagement in children, 176
  GERD, throat pain, throat clearing, and, 91, 92
  irritation-caused muscle tension, 80–81
  mucus and, 76, 77
  swallowing and, 5

inflammation
  from acid reflux/GERD, 66–67, 93
  antihistamine treatment for, 103
  beneficial manifestations of, 144–45
  cortisone treatment for, 144
  from food allergies, 76
  from inhalant allergies, 100
  mucus and, 76–77
  sinusitis and, 94
  throat infections, 80
  of the TMJs, 61
  vocal tract, 133–34
interarytenoid muscle, 23*f*

jaw/jaw tension, 60–64
  bruxism (clenching, grinding), 61–64, 63*f*
  chewing/eating and, 60–61
  do-it-yourself management, 63–64
  influence on singers, 61–62
  management of, 63
  mandible/lower jaw, 60
  masseter muscles, 60
  oral appliances and, 64
  pterygoid muscles, 60
  temporomandibular joint (TMJ), 60–62, 63, 64, 94–95
jazz singing, 21–22, 26, 120*b*

INDEX 197

laryngologists, consulting with, 105–13
 allergy management approach of, 101
 auditory *vs.* visual diagnosis
  preference, 37, 105, 106–7
 cosmetic procedures for singers,
  111–12
 getting recommendations, 113
 for hoarseness, 97, 108–9, 110
 ideal treatment approach, 108
 treatment on tour, 113
 types of available procedures, 109–10
 vocal fold nodules example, 108
larynx, 4–11
 cough mechanism, 6
 description of the untrained larynx,
  6–7
 impact of bruxism, 62
 impact of overpractice, 157
 lowering of, 52
 negative effect of smoking, 143
 protective role of, 4–5
 purposes of changes over time, 176
 role as primary sound generator, 4–5
 role of the upper vocal tract, 12
 swallowing function, 5–6, 7, 52
 upper vocal tract, 11–19
 Valsalva maneuver, 6, 174
 See also larynx, common disorders;
  larynx, structure
larynx, common disorders, 114–28
 blood vessels, vocal fold hemorrhage,
  117–21
 decreased vocal fold movement,
  126–24
 vocal fold cyst, 124*f*, 124–25
 vocal fold nodules, 77, 114–17
 vocal fold polyp, 121, 123*f*
 vocal fold sulcus, 125–26
larynx, structure, 8*f*, 31–36
 Adam's apple, 31–32
 anterior neck contours, 32*f*
 cricoid cartilage, 7, 8*f*, 24, 32*f*, 33–34
 cricothyroid joint, 33–34
 cricothyroid space, 33–34
 depressor muscles, 52
 epiglottis, 5, 7, 8*f*, 36, 176
 front/cross-section view, 8*f*

hyoid bone, 7, 8*f*, 17, 18*f*, 32*f*, 32–33
laryngeal crepitance, 34
laryngeal ventricles, 13–14, 14*f*, 15, 76
levator/depressor muscles, 5–6, 18*f*,
 52–53, 61–62
muscle tension example, 53–54
self-examination of, 31–36
swallowing muscles, 33
thyrohyoid space, 32–33
thyroid cartilage, 7, 8, 23*f*, 24, 31–34,
 32*f*, 68, 154–55, 177
vocal folds, 1, 4, 5–6, 18*f*, 35*f*
lips
 orbicularis oris muscle, 19
 role in voice production, 12, 17, 19, 55
 role in vowel colors, 19
Lombard effect, 49, 152
lungs
 abdominal breathing and, 2
 allergic irritation and, 101–2
 children's development and, 176–77
 coughing and, 6
 impact of smoking, 142–43
 inhalant allergies and, 100
 mucus and, 6, 75
 nose breathing and, 89
 phases of breathing, 3*f*
 thoracic breathing, 2
 total lung capacity, 1

marijuana, 143
medications
 determining the need for, 132–33, 134
 diagnosis challenges, 133
 for hoarseness, cough, excess mucus,
  133
 long-term treatments, 134
 multiple medications, 134
 multiple treatment levels, 133
 short local treatments, 133–34
 for vocal fold nodules, 133
 See also antihistamines; cortisone
  (medical cortisone); decongestants
medications, classes and effects, 135–38
 angiotensin-converting enzyme
  inhibitors, 136
 antihistamines, 103–4, 135

198 INDEX

medications, classes and effects (*cont.*)
  decongestants, 86, 87–88, 102, 103, 135–36
  dermatologic, 137–38
  diuretics, 136
  hormones, 137
  psychiatric, 137
  steroids, 136–37
mindful practice, 157–62
  acquisition of in-the-moment mindfulness, 161–62
  case report/overpracticing, 157–58*b*
  larynx and, 158–59
  learning components of, 160
  methods of improving, 160
  optimal practicing considerations, 158–59
  practicing, anatomic/physiological processes, 159–60
  purposes of practicing, 158, 160–61
  vocal folds and, 157, 159
monitoring the voice, 37–40
  by air conduction, 37–38, 38*f*, 40, 45–47
  by bone conduction, 37–39, 38*f*, 45, 46–47
  importance of hearing the voice, 37
  proprioceptive monitoring of, 39, 49–50
  real time tracking modalities, 40
  role of laryngologists, 37, 101, 180
  role of muscle memory, 39–40
  by singers, 46–47
  visual *vs.* touching/listening, 37
monteleukast, 104, 134
mucus, 75–80
  allergies, respiratory infections, and, 76
  causes of excess mucus, 76–77
  description, 75–76
  elimination diet suggestion, 80
  inadequate mucus, 78
  inflammation and, 77
  medications for excess, 133
  nicotine and, 77
  oral medications, 80
  postnasal drip, 78, 79, 101–2

  relief from, 78–80
  respiratory tract infections and, 76
  throat clearing, 75, 77, 78, 92, 101–2
  too much/too little, 75–76
  yeast infection and, 77
muscle tension/muscle tension dysphonia (MTD), 51–73, 114, 123–24
  ace inhibitors and, 136
  acid reflux/ GERD comparison, 93
  agonist- antagonist muscles, 8, 51, 52
  causes/description of, 52, 54–55, 65, 88, 136
  commonality for singers, 51
  compensation- related, 65
  description, 53–54
  distant/ unconnected, 70–72, 71*b*
  hyoid area tenderness and, 32–33
  influences on the singing voice, 53
  isometric contraction, 52–53
  larynx pull muscles, 53*f*
  Lombard effect and, 49
  lowering of the larynx, 53*f*
  neck and shoulder, 69
  nodules and, 114
  physical posture and, 51, 70
  primo passaggio and, 34–35, 43–44
  repertoire and, 65–66
  secondary, 66–73
  strategies for relieving, 70
  striated *vs.* involuntary muscles, 51
  in teachers, 29
  thoracic scoliosis and, 71*f*
  tongue tie (ankyloglossia) and, 56–57, 58–60
  transient abdominal/ pelvic issues and, 70
  See also jaw/jaw tension; secondary laryngeal tension; tongue/tongue tension
musical theater singing, 21–22
musicians' ear plugs, 49

nasal dryness, 79–80
nasal obstruction, 16*f*, 77, 83–85
  chronic obstruction, 84
  deviated septum, 16*f*, 77
  intermittent blockage, 84

INDEX 199

nasal cavity, description, 83–84
self-diagnosis, 84
snoring, 84
nasal septum, 16–17
deviated septum, 16f, 77
nasal sprays, 6–7, 85, 86–88
nasopharynx, 15, 16–17, 176
natural (reflexive) singing
examples of, 21
vs. trained singing, 21–22, 22t
vibrato comparison, 22t
nicotine, 77, 142–43
nodules, 29
noise pollution, 48–49
nose and sinuses
nasopharynx, 15, 16–17, 176
role in voice production, 15–17

opera singing
repertoire, muscle tension, and, 65–66
singing *fortissimo* challenges, 40
vibrato in, 26
oral antihistamines, 103–4
oral appliances, 63f, 64
oral decongestants, 87, 103, 135–36
orbicularis oris muscle, 19
overpractice problems, 157
oversinging, 49, 90, 146, 159

pharynx, 1
acid reflux and, 91
hypopharynx, 5, 52
lower, 5
nasopharynx, 15, 16–17
natural *vs.* artificial singing, 22t
oropharyngeal resonating cavity, 17
oropharynx, 55–56, 80–81, 82
upper vocal tract location, 11–12, 13–14, 14f
vocal folds and, 36
pitch
chest register muscles and, 24
role of hearing in gauging, 47
role of the vocal folds, 6–7, 11
speaking voice and, 30
vocal folds and, 24
postnasal drip, 78, 79, 101–2

primo passaggio, 24–25, 42–44, 58b, 154, 155b, 156
psychiatric medications, 137
psychotherapy, 64, 110

reinforcement, 68–69
Reinke's edema, 143
Reinke's space, 10f, 10–11, 43, 143
repertoire, muscle tension and, 65–66
resonance/resonators
acoustics of, 12–13
chest *vs.* head voice and, 23
control of harmonic spectrum, 14–15
Helmholtz resonators, 12–13, 13f
laryngeal ventricles, 13–14, 14f, 15, 76
mechanics of, 14–15
performance space, 19–20
resonance, defined, 12
upper vocal tract and, 13–15, 14f, 17
resting tone of muscles, 66–67
rhinitis, 76, 86, 100, 102

secondary laryngeal tension, 66–73
acid reflux/GERD, and, 66–67
laryngitis and, 67
loss of voice and, 67b, 67
resting tone of muscles, 66–67, 68–69
thyrohyoid space palpitation diagnosis, 68
secondo passagio, 24–25, 43
singing voice
chest voice, 22–25, 23f, 27, 116, 155b
head voice, 10f, 22–25, 23f, 29–30, 33–34, 42, 43, 53, 58b, 85, 101–2, 103
untrained "naive" *vs.* trained, 21–22
sinusitis, 85–88
decongestion sprays for, 86, 87–88, 102
herbal remedies for, 87
inhalation of steam for, 86–87
oral decongestants for, 87
rhinitis *vs.,* 76, 86
sinuses, description, 85–86
soprano voice, *spinto vs. soubrette,* 28
speaking voice, 29–30
steroid medications. *See* cortisone
steroid sprays, 103
Sumac, Yma, 27

200 INDEX

sympathetic vibration, 12

teeth, role in voice production, 12, 17, 18, 19, 55
temporomandibular joint (TMJ), 60–62, 63, 64, 94–95
thoracic breathing, 2, 22*t*
thoracic cavity
  abdominal breathing, 2–4, 3*f*, 22*t*
  mechanics of inhalation/exhalation, 2, 3*f*
  thoracic breathing, 1
throat clearing, 75, 77, 78, 92, 101–2
throat discomfort after singing, 88
throat infections, 80–82
  bacterial *vs.* viral, 81
  home remedies, 81–82
thyroid cartilage, 7, 8, 23*f*, 24, 31–34, 68, 154–55, 177
tinnitus, 48, 49–50
tongue tie (ankyloglossia)
  anterior, 59*b*
  case report, 58–60*b*
  laryngeal muscle and, 58*b*
  muscle tension and, 56–57
  tongue tenson and, 59–60*b*
tongue/tongue tension, 55–56
  anterior (free, unattached), 18*f*, 18
  posterior (attached), 17, 18*f*
  role in voice production, 17–19
tonsils/tonsillitis, 80–81, 82–83
  problems in young adults, 82
  removal recommendation, 83
  tonsil stones, 83
topical decongestant sprays, 86, 94, 102
traditional Chinese medicine, 150
trained singing
  vs. natural (reflexive) singing, 21–22, 22*t*
  vs. natural singing, 21, 22*t*

upper vocal tract
  complex effect of resonant spaces, 14–15
  main function of, 12
  moment-by-moment adjustments, 15
  role in a well-trained musical voice, 11–12
  structures of, 13–14, 14*f*

Valsalva maneuver, 6, 174
vibrato
  defined, 26
  musical effect of, 26
  reflexive *vs.* voluntary comparison, 22*t*
  types of, 26
vitamins and minerals
  daily supplements, 129–30
  descriptions, 129
  fat/water soluble, 130
  food *vs.* vitamins, 130
  role in metabolism, 131
  vitamin C, 129–30
  vitamin D, 130
  See also herbal medications
vocal apparatus, 1–20
  larynx, 4–11
  lungs and abdomen, 1–5
vocal fold cyst, 124–25
  comparison to nodules, polyps, 124–25
  description, 124
vocal fold hemorrhage, 90, 117–21, 120*b*
  causes of, 120–21
  comparison to soft tissue injury, 119
  treatment, 121
  visibility of blood vessels, 118*f*
  voice rest for, 121
vocal fold nodules, 77, 114–17
  delayed phonatory onset and, 116
  description/causes, 114–15, 115*f*
  diagnostic method, 116–17
  impact on the voice, 115–16
  initial swellings/"prenodules," 117
  medications for, 133
  mucus and, 77
  muscle tension dysphonia and, 115–16
  spread of hoarseness, 116
  vocal fold polyp comparison, 123–24
  voice rest for, 108, 114–15
vocal fold polyp, 121, 123*f*
  description, 122, 123*f*
  hoarseness and, 121–22
  resolution of, 122–23
  vocal fold hemorrhage and, 121
  vocal nodules comparison, 123–24
  voice rest for, 122–23

INDEX 201

vocal folds, 1, 4
  adductor muscles, 52
  aryepiglottic folds, 5
  chest voice and, 23f
  cortisone treatment for swelling, 145
  coughing and, 6
  decreased movement, 126–27
  false vocal folds, 5, 15, 54
  glissando and, 23–24
  head voice and, 23f
  impact of excess singing, 77
  impact of overpractice, 157
  iPhone visualization of, 35f
  layered structure of, 10f, 10
  lesions, 127–28
  loss of voice and, 67b, 67
  mindful practice and, 157, 159
  mucosal wave and, 9f, 9–10
  muscle tension and, 53–54
  negative effect of smoking, 143
  pitch and, 24
  role in control of pitch, 6–7, 11
  role in sound production, 6–7, 8–10
  true vocal folds, 5
  visibility of blood vessels, 115f
vocal fold sulcus, 125–26
vocal health
  air conduction hearing and, 40
  cortisone and, 149
  diet and, 163–66
  exercise and, 172–75
  glissando test for, 42
  tips for, A1B1–A1B10
vocal ligament, 10
vocalis muscle, 10, 23f, 24
vocal performances, 89, 160, 172, 173,
    175, 182–83
  compared to writing, graphic arts, 182
  exercise and, 172, 173, 175
  learning resources for young singers,
    160
  physical component of, 183
  post-performance vocal rest, 89
  technical mastery requirements, 183
vocal range, 27
  age-related changes in, 27
  defined, 27

  fach and, 27, 28–29, 30
vocal registers, transitions and, 22–25
vocal strain
  description/causes, 88
  laryngeal massage for, 90
  management of, 89–90
  post-singing discomfort, 88
vocal tract
  bone conduction, 37–38, 46–47
  causes of tension within, 73
  impact of irritation of the muscles, 68
  laryngeal massage, 90
  mucus and, 75–76, 78
  muscle tension dysphonia and, 54
  negative effect of smoking, 143
  recovery potential of, 150
  singing naturally and, 21
  tongue/tongue movements, 55
  upper/resonators, processors, 11
voice changes over time, 176–81
  biologic vs. chronologic aging, 177–78
  children, 176
  extrinsic factors, 177–78
  glottic "squeeze," 178–79
  loss of fine neuromuscular control,
    179–80
  men/andropause, testosterone levels,
    178–79
  prolonging good voice advice, 180–81
  pulmonary function changes, 179
  rate/degree of aging, 179
  signs of vocal aging, 178
  teens, 176–77
  vocal muscle atrophy, 178–79
  women/menarche and menopause,
    178
  young adulthood, 177
voice disorders
  diagnosis of, 37, 106
  medical management of, 107
  varied types of treatments, 112
voice production
  Lombard effect and, 48–49, 152
  role of lips, 12, 17, 19, 55
  role of nose and sinuses, 15–17
  role of teeth, 12, 17, 18, 19, 55
  role of the tongue, 12, 17–19

202 INDEX

voice rest, 150–56
  getting back to singing, 154–56
  glissando test/ middle voice tightness, 155b
  for hoarseness, 97, 108–9
  limited/positive effects on swelling, 156
  prolonged rest, 150–51, 154
  reasons for using, 154
  routine rest, 151–53
  for vocal fold hemorrhage, 121
  for vocal fold nodules, 108, 114–15
  for vocal fold polyps, 122–23

voice therapy, 117, 123–26, 145–46, 154
voice types, 28–29

weight/weight loss
  acid reflux, GERD, and, 92, 93, 96
  exercising of portion control, 169
  fat and, 168
  impact of excess, 166–67
  impact of rapid loss, 168
  suggestions for losing, 167–71
  See also diet and nutrition

yoga, 160, 173, 181